"If you are just beginning to lose weight, this book can help you to achieve your goal. If you are making your umpteenth attempt to lose weight, this book can help you to do it right this time. If you have lost weight and are worried about how to maintain your loss, this book can help you to consolidate the changes that brought your eating under your own control. . . .

"I have two copies of Dr. Stuart's book. I keep one in my office and the other in the kitchen. I consult the book when I know that certain crises might arise. Each time that I look for an answer, an answer is sure to be found."

—From the Foreword
by **Jean Nidetch**
Founder, Weight Watchers International, Inc.

**Selected by Book-of-the-Month,
Psychology Today,
and Macmillan book clubs.**

Also by Dr. Richard Stuart

ACT THIN, STAY THIN

NEW WAYS TO LOSE WEIGHT AND KEEP IT OFF

DR. RICHARD B. STUART

PSYCHOLOGICAL DIRECTOR OF
WEIGHT WATCHERS INTERNATIONAL, INC.

FOREWORD

JEAN NIDETCH

FOUNDER
WEIGHT WATCHERS INTERNATIONAL, INC.

A JOVE BOOK

ACT THIN, STAY THIN

A Jove Book / published by arrangement with
W. W. Norton & Company

PRINTING HISTORY
W. W. Norton & Company edition / January 1978
Jove edition (revised) / March 1983
Second printing / May 1984
Third printing / April 1985

ISBN: 0-515-08454-9

Jove books are published by The Berkley Publishing Group,
200 Madison Avenue, New York, N.Y. 10016.
The words "A JOVE BOOK" and the "J" with sunburst
are trademarks belonging to Jove Publications, Inc.

PRINTED IN THE UNITED STATES OF AMERICA

Contents

Foreword

Jean Nidetch
FOUNDER
WEIGHT WATCHERS INTERNATIONAL, INC.

IF YOU ARE just beginning to lose weight, this book can help you to achieve your goal. If you are making your umpteenth attempt to lose weight, this book can help you to do it right this time. If you have lost weight and are worried about how to maintain your loss, this book can help you to consolidate the changes that brought your eating under your own control.

Many of the ideas expressed in this book have already played a major role in the psychological and medical understanding and treatment of obesity. In his Presidential Address before the American Psychosomatic Medicine Society, Dr. Albert Stunkard referred to Dr. Stuart's early work as a "landmark in obesity research." Dr. Stunkard also introduced Dr. Stuart's first book, *Slim Chance in a Fat World*, as "the best book yet written on the control of obesity." These concepts now used in our classes are regarded by many professional observers as the procedures offering most overweight people their best chance for weight loss.

In this new book, Dr. Stuart has greatly expanded the ideas expressed earlier. He offers a comprehensive program for understanding and controlling not only your eating, but also many aspects of your behavior that

bear upon your urge to eat. You will find suggestions
for changing those thoughts and feelings that make
overeating easy and self-control difficult. You will be
shown techniques that can enable you to "reprogram"
forces in your environment that trigger your urge to eat
too much of the wrong food. You will also learn
techniques that you can use successfully to manage hundreds of eating crises and to gain control of your
behavior in other areas.

When Dr. Stuart introduced many of these techniques
to members of Weight Watchers classes through the
Personal Action Plan, members' weight losses improved
dramatically—some by as much as *24 percent!* Some of
the ideas that Dr. Stuart brought to our members were
already in use in our classes: we knew *what* to do
although we were not sure of the scientific background.
Other ideas were new to our members. Most of the ideas
are presented in the context of the research through
which they were derived; knowing where good ideas
come from can help us to keep them working for us.

I have learned a great deal from both the modules
that Dr. Stuart developed for use by members of Weight
Watchers classes and from my careful reading of this
book. I have two copies of Dr. Stuart's book. I keep one
in my office and the other in the kitchen. I consult the
book when I know that certain crises might arise. Each
time that I look for an answer, an answer is sure to be
found.

Selecting this book is a good step in the right direction. When you have the benefit of well-supervised
group support and when you have a professionally
developed food plan to follow, you will have the
elements that can best help you to reach your goal
weight. I wish you every success in your efforts to make
permanent weight control a reality as you achieve a thin,
healthful, and happy life in the years ahead.

Introduction

IN THIS BOOK you will find many new ways to challenge your eating problems by changing aspects of your thoughts, your feelings, your use of your own body, and your social and physical environments. Most of these recommendations have been carefully evaluated in service and research programs in many countries. You are strongly urged to make several changes in each recommended area, and to chart those changes regularly, as suggested. Research has shown that those who make the most changes lose the most weight and those who chart most regularly make the most changes. All of the recommendations will not pay off equally well for you, and some may have to be adapted to your personal needs. To help you in this process, you may wish to consult the research that supports these recommendations. Detailed references to the literature may be found at the back of this book. You may also wish to consult a professional or to join a responsible weight-control program. Either of these steps can help you to develop your personal program for change, and help you to persevere as you meet each new challenge.

Many people have helped to make this book possible. To these people, I would like to offer my sincerest thanks. The book could not have been written were it not for the research of scores of scientists whose efforts provide the basis for the practical program presented here. Albert Lippert, chairman of the board of Weight

Watchers International, had the vision and conviction that allowed many of these ideas to be implemented by being offered to hundreds of thousands of members of Weight Watchers classes. Fred Jaroslow, senior vice-president of Weight Watchers International, supported and guided this effort from conception through fruition. The area directors and franchisees of Weight Watchers International contributed their valuable insights all along the way. Fred Jaroslow and Lenore Lippert read early drafts of the manuscript and made invaluable suggestions for its improvement. My editors, Carol Houck Smith and Eric P. Swenson, helped me to transform some useful ideas that were crudely written in several early drafts into a volume that I hope can help a great many people. Luda Holsgrove took each required rewrite in her stride and turned out clear typed copy without so much as a cross look. Finally, Freida, Jesse, Toby, and Gregory all made work on this book easy by drawing closer together and unselfishly permitting me the time to think, to evaluate, and to write.

R.B.S.
June 1977

ACT THIN, STAY THIN

CHAPTER 1

A New Beginning

HOW MANY TIMES have you gone out for dinner promising yourself that you would eat neither bread nor dessert —only to eat not one but *two* helpings of both? How often have you resolved not to eat one potato chip during the entire late show or one kernel of popcorn at the movies—only to realize later that you stuffed yourself with junk foods you neither wanted nor enjoyed? How often have you promised yourself to start a new diet on Monday—only to remember on Thursday that Monday is long gone?

If you are like most of the readers of this book, you will have had these and similar experiences time and time again. Like the other readers, you have either been heavy for all or most of your life, you have followed the "yo-yo" cycle of periodically gaining and losing from 5 to 60 pounds, or you manage to hover close to, but a little above, your desired weight by expending boundless energy and worry. Finally, you probably have one more thing in common with your fellow readers: you may have tried repeatedly to make the one ineffective weight-control system work for you, without ever being able to maintain your weight loss.

Oh, the details may have been different in your case, but the format was always the same. You talked to friends, perhaps consulted a doctor, or sorted through the dozens of books that promise miraculous weight losses through anything from downing secret formulas to drinking water and holding your breath. Then you selected a diet—perhaps heavy on the steak one time and cabbage or rice the next—and you decided to stick to it come hell or high water. Unfortunately, the high-water mark came early. Whether you followed through for a day, a week, or even a month, the result was always the same: no matter how much weight you lost, you regained it almost as quickly as you took it off.

Most members of the vast army of the weight conscious make the same crucial mistake: when a program fails to bring results they "try and try again." Fortunately there is a much wiser adage to follow: "If at first you don't succeed, analyze what went wrong and try another approach." This could mean reorganizing your thinking about the method that you choose, or it could mean choosing an entirely different approach.

This book offers a way for you to make that new beginning.

What's Different About This Approach?

On Monday you were a "compulsive eater." You were troubled by constant urges to take a bite of this or a taste of that. Your biting and your tasting added up to quite a bit of food and to extra pounds. Then on Tuesday you decided to turn *everything* around. You would curtail your food intake drastically. Same urges: less food to satisfy them. What could you expect for Wednesday besides a new defeat?

You wouldn't try to light a fire on a windy day without shielding the match. Why would you expect to succeed in changing a lifelong pattern of eating without first reducing your urge to eat? As the wind blows out the match, so your urges to eat stifle your ability to control what you eat.

This book will help you to learn *how to manage your urge to eat* while you learn *what* to eat.

It offers a *rational program* for self-management.

It *stems from research* by hundreds of scientists working in scores of laboratories.

And you will be able to *test its effectiveness* in your eating management efforts every single day.

Its goal is to teach you how to *develop self-control*.

Its promise is the opportunity for you to learn freedom from nagging urges to eat night or day for what may be the first time in your adult life.

Self-Control Is a Skill

What we call "self-control" is our ability to achieve the goals we set for ourselves. We generally refer to self-control when the goals are negative, when we plan to deny ourselves the pleasure of eating a snack, or when we plan to force ourselves to complete some unpleasant task. But self-control is much more than that; it includes, as well, every one of the positive goals that we set for ourselves, whether they be finishing a book, learning to play a new game, or painting a beautiful picture.

Oftentimes when we have trouble meeting a personal objective, we explain our failure as the lack of some basic ingredient of character like "willpower," "backbone," or "grim determination." As we blame our ancestors for not giving us the necessary genes or our childhood experiences for not fortifying our will, we swallow hard and make the same mistakes when we try again to accomplish the feat that we feel both nature and upbringing have placed beyond our reach.

The fact is, however, that self-control is a skill that can be learned—in three phases. First, we need a *clear objective*. Reducers should know how much they have to lose and which behaviors they must change to make this happen. Next, we need a *plan for change in small steps.* Reducers who try to shed pounds too quickly suffer prompt regains. Finally, we need *plans for positive action* rather than resolutions about what to stop doing. Reducers must know what they should do to keep themselves on course. Making resolutions about actions to be avoided confuses matters and often leaves them without a plan.

An illustration can help to make this clear. Alice decided for the 27th time in her adult life to lose the extra weight that gave her that roly-poly look. She knew that her weight had been on the rise since her children entered school. She also knew that while her mealtime eating was under control, she often overate when she was bored and lonely in the afternoons or angry at husband George in the evenings. She borrowed a copy of the 600-calorie diet that her friend had used and she set off on a program that would have put the greatest stoic to the test. Overnight, she planned to eliminate from her diet everything that she enjoyed, permitting herself less to eat than would satisfy her five-year-old daughter, Liz. And those afternoon blues and evening rages? Well, they were just her cross to bear.

The results? You guessed it: Alice lasted on her diet exactly four days. Why? She tried to change her eating while the same events that made her bored and angry still took place. She tried to do too much, too soon. And she concentrated on what she should not do rather than setting her sights on positive change. Clearly, knowledge of a few behavioral basics would have stood Alice in good stead.

Some Behavioral Basics

Behavioral basics are what this book is about. If you understand three basic facts about eating behavior, you will be able to understand the objective of all of the recommendations that follow. You must know about hunger and appetite, about appetite chains, and about the many facets of behavior. Each will be explained in turn.

Hunger and Appetite: What's the Source of Your Urge to Eat?

Most of our eating patterns are learned. In this well-nourished land, we teach ourselves to feel "hungry" in a thousand different ways, but this learned "hunger" is actually *appetite*. True hunger is motivated by the physical need for food. It usually does not arise for at least six hours after an adequate feeding, it lasts only a short time before disappearing and it brings with it faintness, loss of concentration, and other bodily signs. Most of us have never experienced hunger. Appetite, on the other hand, appears when our minds reach out for food, not when our bodies signal that food is overdue. Appetite is stimulated by our thoughts, our feelings, proximity to food, habits, and virtually anything that we have learned to associate with food. Almost alone in the animal kingdom, we humans have the privilege of eating to satisfy our appetites, when we are not hungry, and this privilege may one day do us in.[1]

Appetite is one response in a long chain of responses that leads to problem eating. For example, a typical sequence might look like this:

1. Alice feels restless with nothing to do;
2. So she turns on the television when only afternoon "soaps" are on;
3. She watches for a while but her boredom deepens;
4. She looks around for something to distract her and finds the pretzel bowl on the coffee table;
5. Vowing to have three and no more, she lets each pretzel melt in her mouth;
6. Now she's hooked and eats on until the bowl is empty.

Looking closely at this chain of events, it is clear that Alice made one choice after another, each bringing her closer to problem eating. She knows that afternoons are a troubled time for her and at (1) she might have planned to pass the time in more interesting, creative, and productive ways. She knows that soap operas bore her; at (2) she might have phoned a friend, undertaken some long-neglected chore, gone for a walk, or picked up a book instead of turning to TV. Once in the grip of TV stupor, she had another choice at (4): some exercise could have provided distraction and it was not too late to turn to some of the activities that would have been better choices in the first place. Now she comes under the control of a poor decision that she had made days before: she should not have left food in convenient places around the house—should not even have had her favorite snack foods in the house. After eating the three test pretzels at (5), she might have put the bowl away, even thrown out the remaining pretzels. Instead, she left them in easy reach and convenience interacted with boredom to bring on another eating disaster.

This and every other eating experience can thus be analyzed as:

> A SERIES OF CHOICE POINTS
> AT WHICH AT LEAST TWO ACTIONS ARE POSSIBLE:
> ONE CONSTRUCTIVE AND ONE DESTRUCTIVE.

Therefore, every eating urge should be analyzed as a link in a chain of decisions, any one of which can be changed with good result.

Breaking the Appetite Chain

Once you understand the choices that lead to your prudent and imprudent eating, you are in a position to plan constructive action. These plans should *always have at least two stages:*

> FIRST, PLAN TO BREAK THE APPETITE CHAIN
> AT THE EARLIEST POSSIBLE LINK.
> THEN, BE PREPARED WITH BACKUP ACTIONS
> AT LATER POINTS IF THE FIRST PLAN FAILS.

In this way, you give yourself more than one opportunity to rise to the occasion and double your chances of success.

To make the logic of this planning clearer, an analogy may be helpful. Think about the psychologically motivated urge to eat as though it were a river that flows with a definite force. Close to its source, the force of the water is not great but farther downstream it becomes a mighty and irresistible force. It would be a simple matter to cross the river at its source. To do so would probably help you to *avoid* the most serious danger. But something could go amiss during even a simple crossing, so it is a good idea to have a backup plan in mind—a course of action that you can follow should a faster current carry you close to disaster. This would be your way to *escape* the danger that you could not avoid. For example, being ready to scuttle the boat and swim to safety may cost you equipment but not your life.

Deciding where to cross the river and what to do in the event of calamity are moments of truth for the boater. Deciding how to spend her lonely afternoons and what to do to curb her appetite are the moments of truth in Alice's battle for self-control. At a certain point the boater faces a point of no return when all is lost. So, too, does the dieter. Those who succeed in winning their battles with the elements—be they swollen rivers or cresting appetites—plan their first-strike actions carefully and come prepared with backup plans as well. Just knowing the behavioral basic that you should break the chain early and then be ready to act again can start you in the right direction: most of the chapters that follow will help you on your way.

The Need to Take a Broader View

Those who succeed in weight management take action not on one but on many fronts. This was found when a group of 700 former members of Weight Watchers classes were studied to learn the differences between those who did and those who did not maintain their goal weights. All members were offered the same program and all did reach their goal weights. But some maintained their losses and others saw their weights begin to rise. How did the winners differ from the losers in this battle for weight control?

Twice as many maintainers as regainers changed their self-concepts during weight loss: they felt stronger, thought about themselves as "thin at last," and had confidence in their ability to maintain their hard-won losses. The regainers, on the other hand, still thought primarily about their personal weaknesses, considered themselves to be "formerly fat," and doubted their ability to maintain their losses. A different self-concept was therefore one thing that differentiated the winners from the losers.

The maintainers were more likely than the regainers to report that their social life became more active as they lost weight and, as a result, that they considered themselves to be happier. The regainers, on the other hand, were casual in planning meals and in managing their eating environments, two more steps that were squarely in the wrong direction.[2]

In summary, it is a good idea to resist the urge to concentrate all of your energies on a single approach.

Changing the way you *think about yourself* and the challenges that you face is not enough.

Changing the way that you *manage your feelings* is not enough.

Changing the way that you *handle food* in your life space is not enough.

Changing your *interactions with other people* is not enough.

Changing the *way that you use your body* is not enough.

Instead you must do ALL of these and other things as well.

IN A NUTSHELL

Now it's time to sum up. These are the major points in your new beginning.

1. You will have to take an indirect approach, learning to reduce your urge to eat at the same time that you learn new ways of eating.
2. You will have to learn to use your own resources in learning greater skill in self-control.
3. You will have to learn to identify the role of appetite in your urge to eat and then you must learn how to cut that urge.
4. You must learn to identify the choice points in the chain of events that builds your urge to eat.
5. You must learn how to break that chain to avoid some inducement for problem eating and to escape from others that you can't avoid.
6. Finally, be ready to look for opportunities to break the problem-eating chain in many different ways so you can mobilize all of your resources to develop new methods for positive self-control.

If you have attended Weight Watchers classes recently, since I prepared the Personal Action Plan for use by members, you will be familiar with some of the techniques that will be offered. Nevertheless, a number of very useful new techniques have been added to this edition, which has also been brought up to date with the latest Weight Watchers International, Inc., food plan. However, for most readers, this approach will be very different from any that you have followed. If you are in the latter group, the fact that you have read this far probably means that your past efforts have not been richly rewarded. Therefore, it is time for you to make a new beginning.

CHAPTER 2

Putting the <u>Real You</u> in the Picture

BEFORE YOU CAN plan ways to change your eating, you must be able to describe precisely when and how you eat. For example, you must know the hours of the day when your appetite is most likely to get out of hand. You must know the days when your urge to eat is under best control. You must know the times that your self-control is at its peak and the places where your good intentions give way to bad influences. These and dozens of facts like them are essential if you are going to be able to plan successful strategies for controlling what, how much, when, and under what conditions you eat.

The Delusion of the Three Ds

We all share a common frailty: we often confuse what we would have liked to do with what we actually did. For example, we may think that we have followed an eating plan when actually we ate much more than we intended.

Willie, for instance, planned to eat modestly at his sister's Thanksgiving dinner party. He decided in advance that he would pass up sweet potatoes with marshmallows and have fruit instead of pumpkin pie for dessert. Patting himself on the back all the way home, he said, "Oh, what a good boy was I!" But was he? He did have four slices of cranberry bread that he used to soak up that luscious turkey gravy, chestnut stuffing that tasted so good with beans and almonds, and wine to wash down this truly marvelous dinner. The three Ds helped Willy stress what he did right, while allowing him to forget what he did wrong.

The first source of error involves what psychologists call *denial*. Most of us pay much closer attention to those aspects of our own behavior that please us most, and play down our weaknesses. This is all part of a very human process of playing up our positives and playing down our faults.

Denial is a useful defense mechanism because it helps us to maintain a relatively positive image of ourselves. We cannot live happily without it. But when denial becomes excessive, it can lead to self-defeating behavior.[1] So long as Willie denies his eating excesses, how will he ever be able to control them?

Distraction is another source of error. Willie didn't intend to paint his behavior white, but at the dinner party many nice things happened and he was as interested in the warm family feeling that prevailed as in the food that was placed before him. Research has shown that overweight people are more vulnerable to the impact of distraction than those whose weight is normal.[2] And when the distractions are aroused emotions, the effect is all the greater.[3]

The final D that muddles eating recall is *distortion*. Studies have shown that people are more likely to judge their eating intake by what they think they ate than by their eating reality. Expectation reaches out and bends experience out of shape.

When volunteers were fed a liquid diet that they believed to be nutritionally lacking, they felt dissatisfied. But when the very *same* liquid was fed to them in the belief that it contained everything that they needed to be fully satisfied, satisfaction was truly theirs.[4] The same things happen outside the lab. When you decide in advance that something will please, the food will do the job. When you decide that it will not, large quantities can go down the hatch before you reckon that you have had a bite to eat.

How Written Records Can Help

You can overcome the triple threat of denial, distraction, and distortion if you are willing to keep written records of your urges to eat. These records can help you toward reaching two important goals. First, you can obtain an accurate picture of your own food-related feelings. Second, you can actually make strides in bringing these urges under control just because you are aware that they are taking place.[5]

You doubtless have an awareness of when your fancy turns to food, but like many of our beliefs about our own reactions, these beliefs may not reflect reality. You cannot make sound plans for effective behavior change when you start from where you *think* you'd like to be *instead of where you really are*. You also probably slip into patterns of problem eating without realizing that you have thought about or turned to food. Tracking these urges to eat can put you on your guard and help you to see the opportunity to make some choices that turn you away from food.

What to Do

Records of eating urges are helpful to the extent that they are:

1. Specific;
2. Simple; and
3. Kept *before* the eating has taken place.

In Figure 2.1 you will find a specific, simple record to help you to discover with precision when you are nagged by the urge to eat. Begin by drawing a circle around the hour that you wake up, and at the end of the day circle the hour that you retire. Do this in column 1.

In the second column, make note of the level or intensity of your urge to eat during each hour of the day. As you will recall, Chapter 1 pointed out that many of our thoughts of food are motivated by appetite, a psychologically determined urge to eat. Appetite, in turn, tends to be motivated by feelings such as boredom, frustration, depression, and tension, by simply being too close to tempting food, by social pressure to eat, and by a great many other cues for problem eating. Very often when you are exposed to these cues, you will eat *even though your urge to eat is low*. At these times your eating is under the control of external pressures, not internal pulls.

It is important for you to train yourself to differentiate when your eating is motivated by a need for food, when it results from an internally triggered desire to eat, and when it is a response to totally external events. One way to do this is to learn to monitor the strength of your urge to eat and then to analyze when the urge was high and when it was low.

Keeping track of your urges can also help in another way. Just as self-monitoring in general helps to crystalize the fact that you are making a decision about food, assessing your urges before you eat helps to focus the vital question: "Is this food really necessary?" By asking this question *before* instead of after you eat, you can gain one more valuable assist in your effort to bring your eating under strict control. Therefore, use column 2 to record the level of your urge to eat *whether or not you eat during a particular hour*.

Write "0" if you felt no urge to eat.

Write "1" if you feel hunger and believe that it is a

FIGURE 2.1

Urge to Eat Self-Monitoring Chart

Circle Day: Sun.   Mon.   Tues.   Wed.   Thurs.   Fri.   Sat.

(1) Time	(2) Level of Your Urge to Eat	(3) Did You Eat		(4) Planned Action
		Yes	No	
7:00– 8:00				
8:00– 9:00				
9:00–10:00				
10:00–11:00				
11:00–12:00				
12:00– 1:00				
1:00– 2:00				
2:00– 3:00				
3:00– 4:00				
4:00– 5:00				
5:00– 6:00				
6:00– 7:00				
7:00– 8:00				
8:00– 9:00				
9:00–10:00				
10:00–11:00				
11:00–12:00				
12:00– 1:00				
1:00– 7:00				

physically motivated urge to eat. If you ate prescribed amounts of the recommended foods at the proper times, this is likely to occur *only if you have not eaten for at least four hours.*

Write "2" if you feel an urge to eat which is somewhere between a physically and psychologically motivated urge. This will happen during the "gray" hours—a few hours after your last meal but well before your next time to eat arrives.

Write "3" if you feel a mild urge to eat and know that you are not in physical need of food. This could occur either during or after a normal meal. A good test of this condition is to try to shift your attention away from food: if you can readily change your focus, this category applies; but if your thoughts keep returning to food, then it's the next category that fits.

Write "4" if you feel a strong urge to eat and know that you are not in physical need of food. Here you will think of food, try to put the idea out of your mind but find your thoughts constantly wandering back to something to eat.

To make this step easier, take a few minutes to sit back and reflect upon your recent experience. Can you remember the exact feelings of true hunger—perhaps some stomach contractions, a slight weakness in your limbs, or a lack of mental alertness? Now switch to the feeling which you may sometimes have of knowing that you "must" have something to eat even though you know that you have recently had more than enough to eat. These latter feelings are the villains of weight-management efforts and they will be prime targets in your self-management efforts.

Next, turn to column 3. In this column, you are simply asked to check "Yes" if you did eat anything during this hour, and "No" if you ate nothing during this hour.

Column 4 is set aside for a special purpose. You will use it to keep track of your success in taking the behavior change step that is your current focus. For example, in later chapters you will be asked to use this column to make note of the fact that you did take steps

to slow down the rate of your eating, to find alternatives
to eating, to change the events that lead to troublesome
moods, or to make eating a pure experience, among
many, many others. For the present, leave this column
blank. In most of the later chapters, you will learn to
put it to good use.

What Two People Learned About
Their Patterns of Eating

To make clear the use and application of the chart,
let's look at the record that Sandra kept of her Tuesday
eating and what Paul learned about his between-meal
eating all week long.

Sandra is a 37-year-old housewife and she is exactly
37 pounds overweight. If you had asked her to describe
her eating patterns on Monday she would have said: "I
have trouble all the time. I eat from morning till night
and I seem to have *no* control at all." Today, Wednesday, she will give you quite a different answer.
Today she will say: "I do very well until three o'clock in
the afternoon. Then I feel very hungry and eat a snack.
By four, I'm not hungry anymore but I keep on eating
anyway. I have got to give some thought to that three
o'clock snack and I have to plan steps that will help me
to follow my eating plan when my snack satisfies my
hunger."

How did Sandra get so smart, so fast? You can easily
see from her chart in Figure 2.2 that with the exception
of breakfast and lunch at 8:00 and 12:00 respectively,
Sandra ate nothing until 3:00 in the afternoon. At that
time she reported very strong ("level 4") appetite so she
had a snack. Her urge to eat decreased to a lower ("3")
level but she ate nonetheless. She had her dinner at 6:00,
and from 7:00 until bedtime she had no urge to eat.
Given these observations, Sandra can easily zero in on
some eating management planning designed to do two
things: she can plan specific snacks for 3:00 and she can
work out some interesting activities that will keep her

FIGURE 2.2

Sandra's Self-Monitoring Chart

Circle Day: Sun. Mon. Tues. Wed. Thurs. Fri. Sat.

(1) Time	(2) Level of Your Urge to Eat	(3) Did You Eat Yes	No	(4) Planned Action			
7:00– 8:00	0		X				
8:00– 9:00	1	X					
9:00–10:00	0		X				
10:00–11:00	0		X				
11:00–12:00	0		X				
12:00– 1:00	1	X					
1:00– 2:00	0		X				
2:00– 3:00	0		X				
3:00– 4:00	4	X					
4:00– 5:00	4	X					
5:00– 6:00	3		X				
6:00– 7:00	1	X					
7:00– 8:00	0		X				
8:00– 9:00	0		X				
9:00–10:00	0		X				
10:00–11:00	0		X				
11:00–12:00							
12:00– 1:00							
1:00– 7:00							

busy and away from food at 4:00 and 5:00. These specific goals will give her a plan of action and they will help to overcome her general feeling of discouragement about the prospects of achieving her self-control objective.

Paul is in his mid-sixties. He has begun to put on extra weight rather rapidly. After charting for one day —he started on Saturday—he did not find anything unusual. He ate three reasonable meals and had little to eat between meals. Denied a clue from a one-day search, he decided to keep track of his eating for seven days to see if he could find a general pattern. To summarize the seven different charts that he used to monitor his eating every day, Paul developed the form shown in Figure 2.3.

Paul sleeps late on Sunday morning so he did not wake up until 9 A.M. that morning. Therefore he simply drew a dash in the 7:00–8:00 and 8:00–9:00 rows under Sunday column. In the other hours for Sunday he wrote the level of his appetite or hunger for each hour of the day under study. He then filled in blanks for each of the remaining hours.

The summary of his urge-to-eat record tells him when he was and was not strongly preoccupied with food. At the end of each row, he counted up the number of ratings of "2," "3," or "4" he gave himself for each hour of the day throughout the week. At the bottom of each column, he counted up the number of hours during the day that he was plagued by an urge to eat that was at least partly psychologically motivated.

Looking over his chart, can you see where Paul ran into difficulty? Notice that he had no between-meal problems on weekends and almost no problem urges to eat in the evenings. All of his problems seemed to crop up during the day, Monday through Friday. To find an explanation we have to learn a bit more about Paul.

Paul Munson retired from the railroad a little over one year ago. His wife still works in the office and she will not be retiring for another two years. Most of his friends are also still on the job. Therefore he has found himself confronted with idle hours during the day while

FIGURE 2.3

Paul's Week-Long Record

	Sun.	Mon.	Tues.	Wed.	Thurs.	Fri.	Sat.	Total
7:00– 8:00	—	0	0	0	0	0	0	0
8:00– 9:00	—	1	1	1	1	1	1	0
9:00–10:00	1	0	0	0	0	0	0	0
10:00–11:00	0	0	2	0	2	0	0	2
11:00–12:00	0	2	0	2	0	0	0	2
12:00– 1:00	0	1	1	1	1	1	1	0
1:00– 2:00	1	0	0	0	0	0	0	0
2:00– 3:00	0	3	2	2	3	2	0	5
3:00– 4:00	0	4	4	2	2	2	0	5
4:00– 5:00	0	2	3	2	4	4	0	5
5:00– 6:00	0	1	0	0	2	0	0	1
6:00– 7:00	1	0	1	1	1	1	1	0
7:00– 8:00	0	0	0	0	0	0	0	0
8:00– 9:00	0	0	0	0	0	0	0	0
9:00–10:00	0	0	0	2	0	0	2	2
10:00–11:00	0	0	0	0	0	0	0	0
11:00–12:00	—	—	—	—	—	—	—	—
Total	0	4	4	5	5	3	1	—

his wife and friends are at work. He has developed the habit of eating a good deal during these lonely hours, although his eating is under very good control evenings and weekends. To meet the challenge of these idle hours, Paul should make an effort to find activities that will occupy his attention. He could help his wife to run the house. He might clean up his workshop and return to his old hobby of cabinetmaking or he might do volunteer work at a local hospital or school. He could also take advantage of some programs at the public library and might even consider taking a few college courses. Whatever he does, to the extent that he succeeds in constructively and enjoyably occupying his time, he can break the chain which leads to problem eating at a very early link. By knowing exactly when his self-control is put to the severest test, Paul can plan exactly those actions that will strengthen his control.

IN A NUTSHELL

To be successful in self-control, you will need a good idea of just when your urge to eat begins to get out of hand. Unfortunately, your memory of when your thoughts turn to food is likely to be inaccurate: sometimes you deny your feelings; sometimes you experience the urge to eat but are distracted and don't label it as such; and sometimes you simply distort the realities and label appetitive urges as hunger. Use of the written record that is presented as the Urge-To-Eat Self-Monitoring Chart can help you to reach the level of self-discovery that you will need to achieve better self-control. Through this record, you will learn that there are some times when you are truly free from the urge to eat and other times when the urge to eat dominates your life. These are the times when decisions can be made to help you to assert your self-management skills. The following chapters will point the way.

CHAPTER 3

Getting Started
with the Right Ideas

TRUDY IS SO far behind in her work she will never be able to catch up. This leads her to feel tense and overwrought. Thinking that she's failed again and is "all washed up," Trudy decides to have a "pick-me-up": for her, this means two cups of coffee and five slices of toast and jelly. Realizing that she has already eaten too much, she thinks she has proven that she is a failure, feels even worse, and eats more to bolster her faltering ego.

The chain reaction that Trudy just lived through is universal. Our thoughts lead to feelings, our feelings to actions, and our actions to reactions in ourselves and others. For Trudy, a negative thought triggered a negative feeling, and both, in turn, led to negative actions and reactions. If Trudy had thought, instead, that even though she was not finished with her job she had made a good beginning, she might have felt better about herself and worked more instead of turning to food.

Thoughts—feelings—actions—reactions; these are

always the links in our chain of behavior; thus, any success that we have in changing one link of the chain can alter its end result. In this chapter and the next we will deal with techniques that can be used to alter thinking so that our action chains can make a strong beginning. Later chapters will deal with techniques for changing feelings, actions, and even the reactions of others.

Six Errors in Thinking That Most Overeaters Make

Because behavior is part of a chain of events, it is fair to assume that a breakdown in one element of the chain is a symptom of flaws in other elements as well. If you sometimes have difficulty in controlling your urge to eat, then the way you think about food is one source of important clues in breaking the chain of eating urges.

The First Mistake: Incorrect Ideas, Arbitrary Inferences

Unfortunately, there is as much falsehood as truth in popular conceptions about food and weight control.[1] For example, many people believe that they must be hungry if they are to be able to lose weight, that toasting bread cuts its calories, that food eaten at night is more fattening than food eaten during the day, that bread is a greater villain in weight control than meat, or that washing spaghetti removes its starch.

The facts are otherwise. Hunger leads to compensatory overeating; an effective weight-control program that you can follow at home must suppress hunger and allow enough food so that eating is well controlled. Toasting bread removes water but not calories. Gram for gram, meat has more calories and more fat than bread. And washing spaghetti removes its vitamins and not its starch. While some of these are small points, they are indicative of the kinds of errors that many people make.

If you are to plan your diet wisely, you must be able to work from food facts, not fancies. To do this, you would be well advised to consult reputable sources for guidance. Your doctor, the nutrition clinic at your local public health center, or a responsible weight-control organization that has a professionally supervised nutritional program, are good sources of information. You can do many things yourself but nutritional planning should not be a do-it-yourself affair.

The Second Mistake: Dichotomous Thinking

Dr. Aaron Beck of the University of Pennsylvania has spent years studying the kinds of thinking that predispose some people to mental illness, others to good health. He has found that one of the most common mistakes that disturbed people make, and that the sound of mind avoid, is the tendency to think in dichotomies, to categorize life events as *either black or white with never a shade of gray.*[2]

Trudy made this mistake. When her work was not completed she felt *all* bad, and when the job was done she felt *all* good: she never felt a *little* bad or a *little* good. When she was all bad she was beyond redemption; when she was all good she could hardly make a mistake.

Like so many dieters, Trudy considered every extra bite or taste to be a clear and present sign of her weak will. Once her will was weakened she felt that all was lost. Every action, therefore, had the potential to become a stepping stone to disaster because there was no way back from the smallest of mistakes. She sometimes thought that she could "never" change because she would "always" be just the same. Shades of gray were hard for her to see.

Think how much better off Trudy would have been if she were willing to regard herself as human and take small mistakes in stride. When Trudy had an extra slice of toast for breakfast, she considered the day a loss. If the day was Tuesday, the rest of the week was "down the tubes." If the week was the third in that particular month, the next week was lost as well. To avoid the terrible trap of dichotomous thinking, Trudy should have considered her extra slice of toast as a minor setback and gone on to plan constructively for the rest of the day.

Be aware of your either/or thinking. "I am lost—you are saved," "This is a completely bad day—everything is going well today," "I have no willpower—I must be in complete control." Whenever you begin to think in terms of either/or, remember that between black and white there are many shades of gray.

The Third Mistake: Magnification of Errors, Disregard of Positives

Many people also have a tendency to recall and *magnify their errors* and to completely *overlook the positives* in their behavior. On the third day of her weight-control program Trudy ate breakfast, lunch, and dinner as planned. She arranged her activities so as to avoid all snacking between breakfast and lunch and between lunch and dinner. But after dinner, while visiting friends, Trudy ate a slice of her hostess's plum upside-down cake. When she got home that night she felt she had done it again—fallen off the wagon before the trip had barely begun. To console herself, she smeared peanut butter and jelly on a half of a loaf of bread as a midnight snack, even though she almost had to force herself to eat because she was so full.

Trudy might have told herself that she had made a mistake and would have to be more careful in the future. She could have consoled herself by thinking of how well she had done all day long—might even have realized that she had eaten just one and not two slices of plum cake. Rather than magnifying her error and forgetting her achievements, she could have kept her error in perspective.

The Fourth Mistake: Terminal Thinking

The fourth mistake, like the second and third, can point the dieter toward disaster. When Trudy arrived home after the plum cake caper, she wondered *why* she had made a bad mistake. In answering, she told herself that she was "weak," that she had "no willpower," and that she was "born to be fat." Just as night follows day, she concluded that "weak," "willpowerless," and "born to be fat" people have no chance for self-control. The *dead-end language* that she used—"weak," "no willpower," and "born to be fat"—left her paralyzed by terminal thinking with no possible way to overcome the obstacle that she faced.

Instead of thinking about *why* she had gotten into difficulty, Trudy could have pondered *how* she could have handled herself differently. Answers to "why" questions, if they can ever be found, do little more than justify failure and direct attention away from remedies. On the other hand, answers to "how" questions point toward the *process of problem solving*.

The Fifth Mistake: Reversed Thinking

Trudy would like to work on weight control. But she feels down in the dumps and for the past several months has told herself: "When I feel better about myself, then I'll start to do something for me. For now, I'd better not rock the boat." This is a perfect illustration of reversed thinking.

Trudy believes that her mood should change *before* she changes her behavior. But her moods are a *result* of her actions. When she acts positively, she and others react positively. When she acts negatively, she and others react negatively. *Until she changes her behavior, nothing can change her mood.* In her thinking she has reversed the natural sequence of events in the thought-feeling-action-reaction chain, and constructive action is hardly possible.

In reversed thinking, goals are considered in place of the steps that are necessary to reach the goals. It is like trying to complete the roof of a building without having built the walls: there is no chance for success. To un-scramble reversed thoughts, it is necessary to think in terms of first things first, or cause and effect. To feel better, you must change what you do. To change what you do, you must change the way you think. To lose weight, you must change what you eat. To change your use of food, you must manage your urge to eat. With reversed thinking, you back yourself into a box with no way out: straight thinking is the only way for you to plan to reach your goal.

The Sixth and Probably the Worst Mistake: Fatalism

Dr. Albert Ellis founded what has come to be called the Rational-Emotive Approach to therapy. He ob-served that many people share the same general kinds of fatalistic, irrational ideas and that so long as these ideas persist, failure is a foregone conclusion.

Researchers, stimulated by Dr. Ellis's work, con-ducted a survey among several hundred people who had embarked on a weight-reduction program. As pre-dicted, several beliefs about the inevitability of personal failure were widely held. As you read through the statements listed in Figure 3.1, see how many of them have crept into your thinking.

If you checked "Fits Me" for even one of these statements, you have a tendency to create unnecessary problems for yourself. Among the would-be reducers who were tested at the time that they began their weight-loss efforts, those who ultimately succeeded chose an average of 2.3 of these statements; among those who

FIGURE 3.1

Some Common Fatalistic Ideas

Doesn't Fit	Fits Me	
1	2	1. Unless people consistently like and show respect for me, there is something wrong with me.
1	2	2. Because I had eating problems as a child, teenager, or young adult, I can't learn new self-management skills now.
1	2	3. It's my fault when things don't turn out the way that I would like them to be.
1	2	4. It's perfectly natural to turn to food in response to all emotions, from happiness to despair.
1	2	5. Things just happen to me: I can't do anything to improve matters for myself.
1	2	6. It is not fair for anyone to expect me to control my actions whenever I feel upset.
1	2	7. Because I don't expect to succeed at developing better self-control, I don't really expect to do so.
1	2	8. I seem to be jinxed: I'm always the one who has bad luck, who misses out when good things happen.

failed the choice was 4.4. Therefore, fatalistic ideas that you accept at the start of your weight-control efforts can be expected to influence your level of success when your efforts are under way.

Cleaning Up Your Troublesome Ideas

To the extent that you make any of these six mistakes (and we all make some of them some of the time) you will be hindered in your effort to reach your goals, no matter what they might be.

Knowing the more common errors that you might make, you can be alert to their occurrence. When you find yourself slipping into any of these errors, hold an internal dialogue to set your thinking straight. Pretend that you are a member of an international debating team. The other team has just made a case for your negative thought. For example, they have just defended the position that "Every time you feel that you are socially rejected you must resort to food to keep your sanity." Your job is to prove them wrong. You might argue that no one is accepted by everyone and that some rejection is an everyday occurrence. You could also contend that just because someone does not respond positively to you in one encounter they are not necessarily rejecting you. And you could go on to say that they obviously did respond to you with some genuine positive regard even if they were not as overwhelmed by you as you might have hoped. You did handle many aspects of the encounter very nicely and you are learning, now, how to come out farther ahead in the future.

Irrational ideas by definition defy logic. Therefore, one way to get the better of them is to challenge them head-on by attempting to prove them false rather than simply acquiescing in their coercive control of your behavior.

Once you have weakened the strength of the negative statements by refuting them in your own words, the next step is the development of your own positive, alternative messages. To the extent that you confidently expect positive results, you will act in a positive way. To the extent that you act positively, you will enjoy positive outcomes. But merely thinking about positives in general terms is not enough.

Dr. Donald Meichenbaum of the University of Waterloo, who has pioneered in this technology of thought reengineering, found that self-directed statements do little good if they are hollow, overly general sweetness-and-light pronouncements.[3] For example, "Day by Day, in every way, I'm getting better and better" is a statement that does little good. While positive, it does not point the way to any new action. Only when thoughts lead to actions and actions to results can one begin to feel more positively about oneself. Therefore, *the phrases that you use to cue your positive thinking must suggest new things to do*. The following examples illustrate this point:

1. *Irrational thought:* I would like my husband to have dinner alone with me one night each week so that we can have time together without the children. But I'm afraid that he is bored with me and so I'd better not make any new requests of him.
   Constructive thought: My husband probably feels as I do that we are not as close as we used to be. He, too, will like the chance to be alone together one night each week, so I'll suggest that we have dinner after the children have eaten on Friday night.
2. *Irrational thought:* I am not as capable as most of the people I meet so I'd better avoid joining any social groups so that I do not embarrass myself and waste other people's time.
   Constructive thought: All people have different talents. I can do some things better than others and I can gain from being with people who have abilities which I lack. Therefore I'll join the library discussion group, the fund drive for the hospital, or I'll volunteer to work with the Parent-Teacher Association.
3. *Irrational thought:* I cannot control my eating at parties. Everyone sees me make a pig of myself and they think

that I'm awful. So the best thing for me to do is to refuse
invitations so that I can avoid embarrassment.

Constructive thought: I can manage my eating at parties
by having a snack before I leave home and by drinking
only club soda with a twist of lemon while I am there.
Even if I do eat something which is not on my food program, people will not notice because they will be interested in the conversation and other things which are happening. Moreover, I will enjoy being among friends and
will really feel little urge to eat what I am supposed to
avoid because I will feel satisfied by the social contact.

Can you see the irrationality in each of the first
thoughts? Can you see how the constructive thought
creates the condition for positive action? You should
now be ready to purge your thinking of mistaken ideas
whenever they occur, first by refuting them and then by
formulating constructive alternative plans for your own
new actions.

Making Effective Plans

Effective planning is much easier when the ideas that
guide you are sound. To plan effectively you must:

1. Start with facts, not fables;
2. Think in terms of partial success, not total victory or
   defeat;
3. Take a balanced view of yourself, giving your assets
   their full credit while recognizing your liabilities;
4. Think in precise terms about how to take advantage of
   the opportunities posed by challenges rather than pon-
   dering why obstacles have made you powerless; and
5. Plan a course leading from cause to outcome rather than
   expecting results before action.

Many of these errors may have insinuated themselves
into the basic logic of your thoughts. They can be as
subtle as they can be destructive. You can begin to identify them by jotting down a few key words as you think

about the challenges you face at critical times. Just relax and use an uncensored free hand. What are the things that you "know" about the situation? Are they facts or beliefs? Are they true or false? What are the words that you use to describe yourself and the situation? Are they absolute or relative words? As you ponder your relationship to the situation, do you include an accounting of your assets or do you focus entirely on your liabilities? Do you wonder why you got into the mess or do you concentrate instead on how to meet the challenge? Is the horse where it belongs, before the cart? Have you thought in terms of causes leading to desired effects? And have you purged yourself of fatalistic ideas? Self-analysis of this sort can help you clean up faulty thinking that can lead you into one blind alley after another.

A Plan of Action

Planning action requires straight thinking. To think straight you must know:

1. Exactly what you hope to accomplish;
2. Exactly where you stand at the beginning;
3. And what steps you can take to move from where you are to where you want to be.

The goal must be specific. The knowledge of where you are beginning must be precise. And the steps that you plan to take must be small, positive, and all in the right direction. Frank's story shows how it can be done.

Frank knows that he has a problem in managing his eating on weekends. A survey taken among members of Weight Watchers classes revealed that people were more than twice as likely to have trouble managing their eating on weekends as compared with weekdays, and, also, more had difficulty in managing weekend crises than those that cropped up between Monday and Friday. Frank is not alone.

His goal was to follow his food plan all week long, but from 6 P.M. Friday till bedtime Sunday night his motivation was put to the test. He knew exactly what to eat. His self-recording chart told him that middays were his downfall. He analyzed his actions at these times and realized that on weekends he tried to catch up on paperwork from the office and generally worked at the kitchen table. Since he was unhappy that he had to work when he could have been playing, and was surrounded by cues to eat, it is little wonder that he gave in.

Frank sized things up in the following way: "I do well in the evenings and all week long. I have trouble when I work on weekends, and trouble with where I work. Another problem is that when I sit down to work, I never know how much I should accomplish and therefore no matter how much I do, I never feel finished. I also have difficulty in not eating food that I can see and reach. So I had better do two things: I'll decide ahead of time exactly how much work I'll get done, and I'll work in the living room where food is out of sight. If I still have trouble, I'll try to set smaller goals to avoid feeling overwhelmed, and I'll try working in the public library or another place away from home."

Note that Frank didn't try to convince himself that a little extra food wouldn't hurt. He didn't think he was a total failure all week long because weekends were a challenge. He didn't forget his strengths and dwell on his weaknesses. He didn't wonder why it had to be him, and he didn't try to convince himself that he would take constructive action *after* he began to feel more in control. He did chose a goal, learn where he was at the start, and plan small and positive steps, and so he quickly reached his goal.

IN A NUTSHELL

Your ideas are an important starting point for your actions. Positive ideas engender constructive actions; negative ideas lead to self-defeating actions. Your thinking is troubled if what you take for facts are fallacies, if you think in either/or terms that give negatives more weight than positives, and if you stress obstacles instead of opportunities. You're also off the track if you expect results before actions and if you do not move from a knowledge of where you are to where you want to be in a series of small and positive steps.

Jot down the key words that you use when you think about your life at times of stress and try to find positive substitutes for fruitless words and ideas. Also, decide upon specific means for meeting focal challenges so that you always know where you are en route from where you were to where you want to be.

CHAPTER 4

Making Ideas About Yourself Work For You, Not Against You

WE ALL HAVE our own ideas about what we look like and how we behave. The picture of our appearance that we carry about in our mind's eye is our "body image." The notion that we have of the way we act is our "self-concept." Sometimes these pictures are accurate, sometimes less so. Accurate or not, they can give us pleasure or cause us pain. Right or wrong, pleasing or troubling, these ideas about our bodies and ourselves always have a profound impact upon the way that we behave.[1]

Body Image

If we view ourselves as tall, we act as we think tall people should. If we think of ourselves as short, we take on what we believe the manner of short folk to be. If we like our height, we think happily about at least one aspect of ourselves, but if we feel too tall or too short,

34

we constantly stoop to look shorter or stretch to gain an inch or so.

Unfortunately, as a nation, we seem doomed to think that we should be something we're not. In an appearance-conscious culture in which "slim is in" and "fat is ugly," the overweight suffer sorely. Almost as soon as they can talk, children are taught to accept or reject themselves because of the way that they appear. Whether smart or dumb, rich or poor, every child learns that he or she will be accepted if he looks like others and he will be rejected if he looks different. Weight is a very visible difference and one that many a layperson believes to be wholly self-induced. Therefore, many a sad plump child is forced to spend years on the outside looking in.[2] Nor is self-consciousness about weight shed in later years. Few adults avoid the urge to suck in their stomachs or conceal their bulges from the public eye.

If you do not accept your body, there is little chance that you will accept yourself. It is difficult to measure body acceptance objectively, but two researchers did produce a scale that will give you some idea of how you view yourself.[3] A modification of this scale can be found in Figure 4.1.

Along the left side of the figure is a list of personal features. Along the top you will find a list of reactions to these physical characteristics. On the scale of from 1 (strong to moderate desire to change) to 5 (feel fortunate to have it like it is), rate your reaction to each of the aspects of your own body, and then add to find your total score.

A score of 50 indicates perfect body acceptance on this scale, a feat not achieved by anyone in a group of weight losers who were tested. A score of 10 signifies complete rejection of one's sex, age, and body composition. It, too, was not approached in the sample studied. A score above 34 indicates a trend toward body acceptance, with higher scores naturally indicating greater acceptance, while a score of 26 or less indicates a trend toward body rejection. Between 33 and 27, you're indecisive.

FIGURE 4.1

Body Acceptance Scale

Rate each feature of your body by circling the appropriate number that shows the extent to which you would like to change it or are completely satisfied with the feature as it is.

	Strong to moderate desire to change it	Willing to put up with it	No particular feelings about it	Satisfied with it	Feel fortunate to have it
Your sex (male or female)	1	2	3	4	5
Your age	1	2	3	4	5
Facial features	1	2	3	4	5
Complexion	1	2	3	4	5
General shape	1	2	3	4	5

	1	2	3	4	5
Muscle tone and bone structure	1	2	3	4	5
Weight	1	2	3	4	5
Height	1	2	3	4	5
Age	1	2	3	4	5
Sexual characteristics (body hair, breasts, genitals)	1	2	3	4	5

While weight is only one dimension of this scale, it has been found that people who lose weight are likely to improve their self-ratings not only on this feature but on others as well. Weight is thus a pivotal dimension in our current images of how we think we ought to look. For example, a group of overweight adults completed this scale upon joining a weight-control program for the first time. They rated themselves as they saw themselves on Day 1 and at the same time indicated the kinds of ratings which they thought they would select when they reached goal weight. Their projected ratings were an average of 14.5 points better, with satisfaction with sex, age, muscle tone and body structure, and sexual characteristics all showing improvement. Moreover, when they lost an average of only 12 pounds, their average body image score increased 5 points for every 1-point increase in their satisfaction with their weight. In the end, those whose initial scores ranged between 15 and 20 points evaluated themselves at the 30+ level once their weight loss began to improve.

It is important for people to go beyond body-image change into behavioral change as well. As reducers become more satisfied with their body images, they must change their behavior to conform to these images. Some who lose weight maintain a "phantom body size" by continuing to imagine that they still carry about with them the fat they worked so hard to shed. They have been called "thin, fat people"; they are no longer obese, but they remain preoccupied with body size, dwell constantly upon thoughts of food, and even draw pictures of themselves as much heavier than they actually are.[4]

There are many outward behavioral indications of the tendency to preserve the old body image despite a new physical reality. For example, some people continue to go automatically to the size 20-and-over dress racks or to the section of the men's shop offering "portly" sizes, even after they've lost weight. They may continue to walk by shuffling from side to side rather than by thrusting their weight forward by pivoting over the leading leg. (By shuffling from side to side, heavy people can keep their weight distributed on both hips for a greater proportion of their walk time than would be true for a forward-thrust gait. While bone and joint strain is saved, a price is paid in walking speed.) People who fail to adjust their body images to their true proportions also continue to turn slightly rather than walk through doorways in the normal full-front position. They may also hesitate before sitting down as they search for the sturdiest chair in the room. They are likely to decline invitations for social activities, particularly those that require them to wear sports clothes, and when pressed into accepting, they assume the least obtrusive positions in order to avoid calling attention to themselves.

All of these "fat behaviors" are throwbacks to their overweight days. As long as they act as though they were fat in these small ways, the likelihood is great that they will act as fat people do in eating ways as well. Fat behaviors continue as long as fatness is part of one's body image. Therefore it is imperative for all reducers to start early in their efforts to bring body image into line.

There is no vanishing cream that can make a fat body image disappear, just as there is no magic that can hide unsightly flab. You can, however, begin to study your own self-judgments and your own behavior. Do you tend to think of yourself as fat? Do you begin to size up your appearance by checking first to see whether you are thin and trim? Do you think about others first in terms of weight and then in terms of other characteristics?

Any time that you become aware of these telltale signs of fatness in your body image, repeat the thought but replace "fat" with "thin." If you think of yourself as fat, repeat the thought with you as "thinning." Choose other aspects of your appearance for special note as you dress or prepare to leave the house. And when you think of others, concentrate on how they behave instead of on their good looks. Anything that you can do to train yourself to shift your attention away from a preoc-

cupation with excess weight can work to your advantage
in giving you a better balanced, thinner body image.

Self-Control

Your behavior is the key to the way others know you
and the way that you understand yourself. As far as
other people are concerned, *you are what you do.* After
an initial meeting, when your appearance can play a
role, others will evaluate you mostly in terms of the way
that you act. Act in a way that others consider positive
and you will be seen in a positive light; act negatively
and the evaluation will change.

Your assessment of yourself is very much more com-
plicated, however. While others may know you in only
one situation, you know yourself in many. While others
see only what you do, you know what you intended to
do and the alternatives that you rejected in selecting a
course of action. Others have a relatively simple task in
deciding who you are and what can be expected from
you. For you, the job is huge if only because you have
so many of the pieces of that very complex puzzle that
makes you what you are.

We work hard at developing a concept of ourselves
and we know that this concept will be ever-changing.
Most of us have a tendency to be a little kinder in our
judgments about ourselves than others might tend to be,
but at times we can be harsher. Right or wrong, kind or
cruel, our concepts of ourselves strongly influence
everything we do.

Norman knows that he "can't" resist chocolate and
Susan knows that she has "never" controlled her eating at parties. What Norman "can't" do and Susan
"never" did become the ground plans for the future
because words like "can't" and "never" are almost
sure to become self-fulfilling prophesies.

Fortunately, we can weaken this link in the chain of

self-destructive behavior: we can change the messages that we give ourselves and thereby help to change the course of our future behavior. To do this, we must change what we think *and* what we do. We must begin to give ourselves positive messages, but these messages will ring true only if we change our behavior as well.

Take the case of a woman whom we will call Jane. She was a bridge player and snacking was part of her game. She knew that she "always had to eat to keep her tension down." One night she decided that she could change that old familiar tune. Instead of telling herself that she *couldn't* manage her eating while sitting South, she told herself that she *could and would*. To back this up, she had a small snack before she went off to the game and asked that the pretzels and nuts be placed within North's reach and out of hers. She had a nut or two that first night but much less than ever before, and at the next bridge game she was even better.

When Jane began to think back over her old "I can't" statements, she realized that she was really saying "I won't." Then she realized that "I won't" could become "I will." When she turned this corner, she began her first real change toward better self-control by changing the person she thought she was.

It is helpful for you to start your weight control efforts with a knowledge of how you truly size up your self-control potential. Are you in the "I have never had and never can have power to manage my own behavior" camp? Or do you realize that you do have the power to control your own fate? The Self-Control Potential Scale in Figure 4.2 will help you to learn about this very important dimension of your self-concept.

The items in this scale are developed from the original work of one American and two Canadian psychologists.[5] The scale has proven useful in predicting who will and who will not maintain their goal weights once extra pounds are lost. If you know that you tend to take an "I can't" point of view at the start of your program, you can concentrate on developing your "I will" potential; in that way you can increase the chances that you will

FIGURE 4.2

Self-Control Potential Scale

Each of the following twelve items has two alternatives. Please read both alternatives carefully and circle the letter of the item which best characterizes the way in which you have felt during the past two weeks. Please be sure to circle one of the alternatives in every item.

---

1. A   My behavior is frequently determined by other influential people.

   B   I always feel in control of what I am doing.

---

2. A   There are moments when I cannot constrain my emotions and keep them in check.

   B   When I put my mind to it I can constrain my emotions.

---

3. A   Many times I feel that I might just as well decide what to do by flipping a coin.

   B   In most cases I do not depend on luck when I decide to do something.

---

4. A   People cannot always hold back their personal desires: they will behave out of impulse.

   B   If they want to, people can always control their immediate wishes, and not let these motives determine their total behavior.

---

5. A   In this world I am affected by social forces which I neither control nor understand.

   B   It is easy for me to avoid and function independently of any social forces that may attempt to have control over me.

---

6. A   Most of my present behavior is determined by genetics and by my experience when a very young infant.

   B   I have the power to work hard enough to be able to achieve my major objectives in life.

7.	A	I frequently find that when certain things happen to me I cannot restrain my reaction.
	B	Self-regulation of one's behavior is always possible.
8.	A	I feel that I must yield to social pressure because I am very uncomfortable when I go against the wishes of others.
	B	I generally feel that it is more important to act on my own good judgment than to do what others advise me to do.
9.	A	Even if I try not to submit, I often find I cannot control myself from some of the enticements in life such as overeating or drinking.
	B	When I make my mind up, I cannot always resist temptation and keep control of my behavior.
10.	A	I often realize that despite my best efforts some outcomes seem to happen as if fate planned it that way.
	B	The misfortunes and successes I have had were the direct result of my behavior.
11.	A	Something I cannot do is have complete mastery over all my behavioral tendencies.
	B	Although sometimes it is difficult, I can always willfully restrain my immediate behavior.
12.	A	I have no control over the way that I feel, the things that I think, or the way that I act upon my feelings and thoughts.
	B	I can control my thoughts and behavior and therefore I can control the way that I feel most of the time.

both lose weight *and* maintain the loss once it has been achieved.

Please read the instructions on the scale and choose one of each pair of alternatives. In scoring the scale, "A" and "B" items have different values. Each "A" item counts 1 point and each "B" item is valued at 2 points. When you have added up your score, you will find that the possible range is from 12 to 24 points. A score of 12 indicates a complete lack of faith in your ability to manage your own behavior because you see your impulses, fate, and other people all pulling the strings that control your movements. On the other hand, a score of 24 indicates that you view yourself as fully in control of your own actions at all times.

The Self-Control Potential Scale consists of three sets of items. Items numbered 2, 4, 7, 9, 11, and 12 refer to the extent to which you feel that you are in control of your own thoughts, feelings, impulses, and actions. Low scores on these items suggest that you feel relatively powerless to manage forces within yourself while high scores indicate a feeling of self-mastery. Items 1, 5, and 8 measure the extent to which you feel that your behavior is under the control of other people, while Items 3, 6, and 10 assess the extent to which you consider yourself to be in the hands of fate.

If you have chosen items in the first series that indicate that you feel you are in control, you are likely to choose few items in the final two series attributing control of your behavior to outside forces. If you checked low-self-control items, you might or might not have checked items that put your behavior in the hands of others or of fate because you might feel that your actions are under the influence of the deeper recesses of your own being.

To the extent that you accept responsibility for your own actions, you will take steps to improve your self-management behavior. However, if you feel that you do not have control, you will be much less likely to do what you should do in order to accomplish your goals. If you have recorded a low score on these items, take special precautions to overcome your initial doubts about your abilities as you approach the recommendations in this book. Furthermore, be sure to interpret every success, no matter how small, as proof that an "I can't" statement can become an "I can, I will, I did!" statement.

Some Steps to Take

There is no guarantee either that weight will be lost or the loss maintained when self-concept is changed. But the probability is great that the process will neither be started nor sustained unless positive changes in self-regard are accomplished. This means that you must change the persistent wallpaper of your consciousness— the kinds of things that you tell yourself about yourself from morning to night every day of your life. You have had many years of practice for your negative thoughts so you must expect to work very consistently to change these crucial ideas about yourself. The success of your efforts depends upon the *seriousness* with which you approach the task and your *consistency* in following through.

First, you have to think about the most negative things you tell yourself. Norman told himself that he was a "chocolate freak, who could never say no to a piece of candy." Susan told herself that she "couldn't resist canapés and cakes at parties." Jane told herself that "for me, bridge decks and peanuts go hand in hand." Toby knew that he was "born to be fat," Natalie that she was "still a fat mind in a slimming body," and Marilyn that her "appetite was in the driver's seat." What are the two or three *negative* self-statements that you make to yourself time and time again every single day? Write them in the spaces below:

1. _____
2. _____
3. _____

Now go back over these negative messages and change them into positive self-statements. Norman can tell himself: "I can control my eating candy as well as anyone else." Susan can say: "By having a snack before the party, I can keep from eating anything while I am there." Jane can tell herself that her "interest is card play and not junk foods," Toby that "thin is a set of behaviors that he has already begun to develop," Natalie that she has a "new thin sense of self," and Marilyn that she has "her urges to eat on the run." In each instance, the message is simple, easy to remember, and to the point. Above all, each one is concerned with what can and will happen, and weakens old ideas about what can't or won't.

Looking back over your original negatives, rewrite them now as positive self-statements.

1. _____
2. _____
3. _____

There are two different sets of times that you should select to begin making these statements to yourself.[6]

First, every time that you catch yourself making a negative statement in that inner dialogue we always carry on within ourselves, silently order yourself to "Stop that nonsense!" and then repeat the positive message.

Second, plan to repeat these important positive messages to yourself at regular times every single day. For example, if you drive to work, make a positive self-statement every time that you stop for a red light. If you do something several times each day like washing dishes or straightening your desk, repeat the positive message before you do the chore. Or if you look at your wrist-watch several times each day, try to train yourself to repeat a positive self-statement every time you do. List below the times and situations when you will choose to cue your new self-statements every single day:

I can think about other things other than sweets.

Positive Self Statements

I can resist eating sweets & can choose To eat them when _I_ want to.

I don't have to have ~~sweets~~ Choc. everyday

I'm _not_ a failure. I do ~~many~~ things wel

I can do it.

It's possible to be & remain in control.

You
really goofed this time muffed up
original negative
I'm so depressed
I can't resist sweets

I have to have _some_
chocolate every day

I'm a failure
It's no use
I'll never do it

It's too hard to be

in control

all I ever do is think
about sweets

<u>IN the morning</u> –
 I'm not a failure
 I do <u>many</u> things well

<u>IN the afternoon</u>
 It is possible to <u>be</u> &
 <u>remain</u> in control

<u>in the evening</u>
 I <u>can</u> do it

In the morning: _____

In the afternoon: _____

In the evening: _____

Only by interrupting the thought chains that begin with self-criticism and by developing high-strength habits of positive self-statement can you begin to be successful in changing your self-concept in a way that keeps pace with your slimming self.

Any task worth doing is worth counting. As a way to help you to remember to think kindly about yourself, and as a way of helping you to assess the consistency with which you have applied yourself to this vital self-redevelopment task, use the left-hand segment of the fourth column of the Self-Monitoring Chart on page 27 to keep track of the times that you do remember to reprogram your concept of you. If you change bad messages into good and restate the positive messages inwardly ten or twelve times each day, you will be well on the way toward bringing your self-fulfilling prophesies into line with your personal goals for change.

IN A NUTSHELL

We all have inner ideas about our bodies and about our behavior. Whether these ideas are right or wrong, pleasing or painful, they do influence our behavior. If we think of our bodies as fat and ourselves as weak, we are very likely to perpetuate self-defeating behaviors. On the other hand, if we can change fat body images to thin ones at the proper time, and replace doubts about our ability to exercise self-control with confidence in our abilities as our strength in self-control grows, we have a much stronger chance of accomplishing our behavior change objectives. In this chapter you have had an opportunity to size up your body image and your belief in your potential for self-control. You have been offered ways in which you can improve your scores on both important dimensions; as your body begins to shed its weight, your body image will be slimming, too. Even before your shape begins to make visible change, start to rethink your ideas about your own behavior so that you think of yourself as "thin behaving" and stop cueing yourself to act as though you were doomed to everlasting fatness.

CHAPTER 5

Getting the Goods
on Your Pantry Shelves

THE DIET OF the average American is changing—and changing fast. Since 1935, the typical adult in this country has increased his or her consumption of red meat by some 50 percent, to 187 pounds annually. We have more than tripled our poultry consumption to 50 pounds per year. We eat more than twice as much cheese as we did forty years ago (some 15 pounds per person per year). We eat about the same number of eggs per year (285), put away about the same amount of sugar (100 pounds), and wash it all down with about the same amount of coffee (14 pounds). At the same time, our intake of fresh vegetables has declined by close to 15 percent, we drink about a third less milk than was consumed in the past, and we eat over 40 percent less fruit.[1] In place of reaching for a carrot, a glass of milk, or an apple, our hands fall instead on pastries (up 70 percent), soft drinks (up 80 percent), and "munchie" foods like potato chips (up over 85 percent).[2] While we talk more and more about healthful eating, we are turning away from fresh nutritious food to processed foods with empty calories. So great is the impact of this change that the U.S. Department of Agriculture has found that over half of all Americans now have inadequate diets, up 10 percent in a single decade.

If our incomes are small, about thirty cents out of every dollar spend goes to pay for food. If we are more fortunate and find ourselves with more generous incomes, we spend about twenty-one cents of each dollar earned for food. It seems as though with each increase in food prices, we become less concerned with the declining nutritional value of the foods that we eat. What has helped to blind our vision so?

Technology on the March

Prior to World War II, foods were processed primarily to improve their shelf life and food advertising was limited basically to print ads advising consumers about the price and availability of foods. During the war, technologists were called upon to produce new methods and materials at an unprecedented rate. Transportation, munitions, human engineering, and communication technologies produced innovations with unprecedented speed and dependability. One of the challenges posed by the war was the need to bring preserved foods to servicemen in the field in easily consumed individual portions. Rising to the challenge, the food industry developed the infamous "C" and "K" rations which both assured the survival of hundreds of thousands of GIs and dulled their palates for years to come.

After the war, we had surpluses of manpower and technology. It did not take long to find ways of putting both into action again. The workers and the machines that brought hardtack and beef jerky to the servicemen were employed to bring convenience foods into the homes, offices, and factories of America. Technology was used to devise new forms for food that would have staggered the imagination of the chief cook and bottle washer on Buck Rogers's interplanetary space rocket.

Where Has All This Gotten Us?

We eat about the same number of calories today as we did in 1940 but the nutritional value of this food has suffered a steady decline since the end of World War II.[3]

Several technologies have played crucial roles in this change. The technology of food processing has developed an unprecedented array of new foods and new forms of familiar foods. The technology of advertising has had a large impact upon changing public attitudes toward these foods. And the technology of marketing has worked to lower buyer resistance in the actual marketplace. Consumers ultimately pass judgment on the success of these technologies and their vote must be seen as one of resounding approval as they buy increasing quantities of the new foods and shrinking quantities of the old. "Synthetic" seems more valued than "natural," and "convenience" has come to dominate "economical" as values among the food buying public.

Unfortunately, many of these new foods are made palatable by the addition of unprecedented amounts of sugars and fats, and the packagers, advertisers, and marketers have become so skilled at their trade that the food-buying public is bombarded to buy more than they need—and more than they should have. Food on the shelf cries out to be eaten and, therefore, it is important for weight-conscious people to develop the skill necessary to buy what they need and only what they need.

TV and the Urge to Act

Which tablets absorb over forty-seven times their weight in acid? Which bread builds bodies twelve ways? Which mouthwash tastes bitter but fights bacteria? Nearly everyone over the age of twelve can answer these and dozens of questions like them. We know more about the absorptive capacity of some antacids than about the caloric value of fat. We know more about the supposed virtues of some breads than about the importance of fruits and vegetables. And we know more about how to keep our breath smelling sweet than about how to choose foods wisely.

All of us have learned these tidbits in the privacy and comfort of our own living rooms while watching one of the some 122,000,000 television sets that carry their message into 90 percent of the homes in America.[4]

It has been estimated that children view between 8,580 and 13,260 televised commercials per year, or an average of over 100 running hours of commercial messages. During what is believed to be "kiddie prime time," advertising is limited to 9.5 minutes per hour on Saturday and Sunday mornings and to 12 minutes per hour on weekday mornings. Also, during these hours, advertisements urging children to ask their parents to buy certain products are prohibited and stations are prevented from running ads in which the cartoon heroes of adjacent programs are used to hawk a product. But children watch many hours of television during the afternoon and early evening hours and no such protections are afforded during these important times. Children are thus unprotected during all but about 10 percent of their TV-viewing time.

Repeated time and time again, and presented in picture and sound that often competes successfully with the program itself, televised commercials have a great capacity to influence. They can help to disseminate an understanding of nutritional principles and to market healthful and nutritious foods. Or they can promote the consumption of foods which are as destructive in their effects as they are costly in price. Unfortunately, it is clear which end comes out on top in the choice between education and commercialism.

A look at the list of products that are offered to children by the clowns and cartoon figures who prance across the Sunday morning TV screen is frightening indeed. Consumer activist Robert Choate took notes one Sunday morning in his hometown, finding that on children's programs all of the products advertised between 10 A.M. and noon were empty-calorie, highly sweetened junk foods.[5] The child who fell victim to all of these ads would spend his adolescence in the dentist's chair if he were not too fat to make the trip to the dentist's office. Clearly, the foods sold to children by TV stations in Choate's hometown rank high on the list of nutritional bombshells.

According to the *Broadcast Advertisers Report,* during the first nine months of 1975, and on the three commercial networks only, there were:

8,166 cereal commercials
4,083 ads for candy and chewing gum
3,208 ads touting shortening and cooking oils
3,024 soft drink commercials and
2,129 cookie and cracker ads

During the same time, you could count on one hand the number of national ads for fruits other than oranges and vegetables of any description.

Many of the ads which are aired on TV are aimed primarily to child viewers. A review of which ads are slotted during children's viewing times and which during adult hours is informative. The following figures were also adapted from the *Broadcast Advertisers Report:*

Product	Percent Sucrose	Number Weekend Broadcast	Number Total Broadcast	Percent Weekend Broadcast
Cereal A	55.1	279	334	83.53
Cereal B	50.0	141	143	98.60
Cereal C	48.8	279	288	96.88
Cereal D	46.6	121	122	99.18
Cereal E	45.9	187	201	93.03
Cereal F	10.6	37	259	14.29
Cereal G	8.1	0	219	0
Cereal H	4.4	0	260	0
Cereal I	4.1	0	278	0

Notice that the cereals with the highest level of sucrose (refined sugar) are those with an overwhelming percentage of their ads scheduled during prime time for the kiddies, while the cereals with modest sugar content are virtually hidden from children's view. What does this tell children about which foods are good to eat? What will they ask their mothers to buy? And what impact will eating presweetened cereals, candy, and soft drinks have upon their waistlines and their health forty, fifty, or sixty years later?

Children are not alone as targets of the food advertisers. According to a summary in *Advertising Age,* during 1973, large food manufacturers spent as much as $180 million on advertising. Close to 90 percent of these expenditures were allocated to television by these major advertisers and by others who help to push food advertising past $1.5 billion per year.

Some of this money is used to fund ads that present simple facts about foods that are offered for sale. But some of the money goes into ballyhoo ads that by inference and innuendo try to represent a product as something which it is not. The goal of most of these ads is at best to inform consumers about the availability of services and goods that might not otherwise come to their attention. At their worst, however, unscrupulous advertisers urge consumers to make purchases that otherwise knowledgeable buyers would fail to make.[6]

The common threads in these legal, yet deceptive, are juxtaposition and inference that lead consumers to false ideas. The following is a listing of several different types of deception:

1. *Virtue by Association Ads.* The background for these commercials is the information that consumers tend to associate certain virtues with certain product characteristics. For example, if it is known that consumers believe that athletes gain their strength by eating certain foods, the suggestion that athletes eat a particular product activates an expectation that eating that product will lead to athletic prowess.

2. *Incomplete Statements.* How often have TV announcers proclaimed that "three out of five doctors recommend brand X diet supplement pills?" We, naturally, assume that a majority of physicians endorses the supplement in question. But are the doctors physicians? biochemists? doctors of divinity? or doctors of veterinary medicine? Under what conditions do they recommend the pill? For what disorders? Against which alternative? And did literally three out of five make the recommendation or was it 30 out of 50 or 3,000 out of 5,000? Clearly the "three out of five" statement is intended to reach far beyond the simple meaning of the words.

3. *Incomplete Remedy Ads.* "Buy XYZ formula and lose pounds in hours, inches in days!" What's implied? That XYZ formula alone will produce dramatic weight-loss results. But read the fine print on the package liner when the magic elixir arrives: it also requires a 600-calorie-per-day diet and two hours of hearty exercise every day. Then ponder the situation: the diet and the exercise alone can produce the weight loss—Dr. X's magic potion is harmless (we hope) and useless (we know) icing on the cake. The same kind of logic is found in ads that promise 50 percent of the minimum daily requirements of certain nutrients when one cup of "Breakfast Delight" is included with four ounces of orange juice and a glass of milk every morning. Check the tables and what do you learn: the nutrients are in the orange juice and milk!

4. *Fool's Gold Ads.* These are the ads urging consumers to buy a product in order to take advantage of its fun-

damental element. "Buy Wonder Vitamins and give
your vision a boost with retinol!" Retinol does help to
improve vision but it is another name for vitamin A₁
and it is found in virtually every multi-vitamin capsule
sold over the counter.

5. *Food Is Love Ads.* This ad preys upon human frailty.
We all want to be loved. If we are parents, we want the
affection and respect of our children. If we are spouses,
we want our husbands and wives to know that we care.
If we are friends and relatives, we want them to know
that we are wise and gracious. Therefore, many, many
foods are sold with the following scenario:

Junior rushes into the house after a long day at
school: "Hey Mom," he shouts, "I'm home. What ya
got to eat?"

Mom reaches into the cupboard and comes out with
an instant treat.

"*Wow!*" says Junior. "At Billy's we never get things
as good as this!"

Moral of the story: If you want to outdo Billy's Mom
and score high on your child's hit parade, buy a treat
which he should probably never eat.

The key to these ads is thus the inference that some
positive social feelings are tied to serving a particular
foodstuff, an inference which is as absurd as it is
destructive.

All of us, old and young, white and black, male and
female, rich and poor, fat and skinny—yes, all of us
are vulnerable to the ads. Unfortunately, some of us are
more vulnerable than others, especially the young, the
less educated, and, where food ads are concerned, the
overweight as well.[7]

The overweight were shown to be vulnerable to the
lure of ads in a simple experiment. Researchers at the
University of California at Davis showed some food
slides to groups of heavy and normal-weight subjects
and slides of pretty scenery to other subjects of varying
weight. All subjects were then asked to rate the taste of
crackers and to indicate whether or not they would pur-

chase packages of the crackers which they were tasting. You guessed it: while normal-weight subjects did not seem to be influenced by the slide show, overweight subjects seemed willing to buy more types of crackers after having been shown food slides than after having been shown scenery slides.[8]

The Plot Thickens

Food packaging is big business. In 1971, the average American made use of 591 pounds of food-packaging material. Forty-seven percent of all paper products, 14 percent of the national aluminum production, 75 percent of our glass output, and 29 percent of the plastics go into materials used to package food. All of this is quickly processed by the family and becomes one-third of all household refuse, the largest single component of municipal waste-handling systems.[9]

Packaging, of course, does help to preserve food and to protect it from damage. But it has two other very important functions. It facilitates handling of foodstuffs by market managers who can cut labor costs when cream cheese comes foil-wrapped and placed in cardboard boxes (rather than in one solid brick needing cutting) or when tomatoes come nestled in cellophane-wrapped plastic trays (rather than being displayed loose on large counters). While serving these utilitarian functions, the packaging in which food is marketed is also a form of point-of-sale advertising. Its purpose is to attract attention.

Food packagers spend large sums of money in order to determine the best way to present their wares. Some cookies have been found to have great eye appeal and are resistant to breakage and easily stacked; they are sold in see-through packages. Other cookies would look attractive if they were not so fragile and if they held their positions in columns; their pictures are printed on wrappers. And still others are not very interesting to look at; they are decked out in packages with fancy lettering but no likeness.

The colors of the wrappers are scientifically chosen and the choice of the brand name and the wording of the package label are both as carefully test-marketed as is the food itself.

All decked out in attractive garb, the product is then passed along to the market manager who has some very important decisions to make. Products that are displayed between waist and eye level naturally attract more buyer interest than do those that are on low or high shelves. Staples, the items that customers will seek out, can be placed where they are more difficult to see, with the most visible display area assigned to those products for which the store manager would like to attract buyer interest. Other foods are more easily seen in open display cases, so considerable energy is consumed by keeping frozen foods frozen and chilled foods chilly in refrigeration units, the doors of which are constantly open—a feat that astounds utility-bill-paying home-owners.

Some surplus and hard-to-market items are placed in sale bins at the ends of aisles so that customers are certain to see them as they round the bend en route from fruit juices to breakfast cereals. Other items are placed in racks adjacent to the lines in which customers must stand while waiting to pay for their purchases. These are often items with appeal to children, who nag their parents to make an unnecessary purchase under threat of a row that will bring disgrace to one and all. At other times, items which shoppers would normally pass up, but which they might drop into their carts when given several minutes of boredom and inactivity, are put on display before customers in checkout lines.

Such, then, is the industry that has developed to manufacture need. Advertising seeks to condition favorable responses to products, from techniques as simply as merely repeating brand names so that they are recognized in stores, through the communication of information which can aid intelligent selection of the product, to ads which intentionally mislead through implication or outright lie. Some advertising also seeks to build demand by programming children to ask for products which they do not need and would often be better off not having. Meanwhile, the food packagers and store managers are making ready to close the sale by decking foodstuffs out in fancy wrappers and by arranging displays which all but guide the hand to discretionary (read *unnecessary*) merchandise.

How to Evade the Shopping Traps

The unwary consumer who watches his or her television set in earnest and who goes unprepared into the marketplace is a "sitting duck." Armed with the clichés of the ad men, still hearing junior's request for What-Not Honey Flakes, and scanning the shelves for "good" buys, the unprepared shopper is very likely to shell out dollar upon dollar for unnecessary food, leading to pound upon pound of extra fat. On the other hand, the wary shopper who analyzes the commercial messages and who prepares for the foray into the marketplace has a much better chance of arriving home with only the items which are needed.

The key to successful shopping is to apply the cardinal principle that has been used throughout this book: *break the chain at the earliest possible point, and be ready with an escape plan if avoidance fails.*

- The buying chain starts with the manufacture of demand by advertising: try to resist the entrapment of ads.
- The chain continues when demand for items is voiced by other family members: try to resist acceding to requests which you consider unwise.
- The chain is lengthened when the decision is made to go forth to the market: make certain that this decision is made at the best moment for you.
- The chain ends in the store as you make your purchases:

arm yourself so that you steer clear of the snares set by
the packagers and market managers.

Here, as elsewhere, the chain is strong and it can be
broken only with careful advance planning. Let's
explore ways to break the chain at each of its critical
points.

1. Build Your Resistance to Promotions of Food on TV

As in love and war, the best defense against the on-
slaught of TV is a good offense. It is also essential to
have a good defense in reserve.

As an offense, *cut down the number of food commercials to which you and your family are exposed
every week*. This can be done by a range of different
stratagems which vary in strength.

A. For a start, try to reduce your TV viewing time. Watching
television is about as passive a pastime as humankind has
conceived. It requires no activity and little if any imagination and/or intellectual ability. Long hours of televiewing
can fatten the body and dull the senses. Therefore, finding
activities that provide more stimulation can both help to
flatten the belly and sharpen the mind.

B. If TV's your affliction, try to vary the programs you watch
by turning in to at least some noncommercial broadcasts.
Many cities now have educational television stations where
some of the best broadcast fare can be found.

C. When commercial television is your choice, plan in
advance activities which you will pursue during the typi-
cally two-minute program interruptions. You could, for
example, turn the TV volume down and

    (1) Converse with friends and family members—you'd
be surprised how much family business can be discussed in nine to fifteen minutes of every TV hour;

    (2) Begin a solitary pastime such as crossword puzzles, a
craft project, or a jigsaw puzzle, or start a family
game in which each member of the family takes one
to two turns during each break;

(3) Use the commercial time to get a little exercise by climbing up and down a flight of stairs once or twice or strolling around the house. The activity can help to pep you up while shielding you from the commercial.

D. When you do watch commercials, try to psych them out. For example, on a typical evening you might see ads for many of the following items:

A presweetened cereal _____

A snack food _____

A soft drink _____

A cleaning compound _____

A toiletry _____

An automobile or _____

An appliance _____

Watch the ads with a critical eye and, with pencil in hand, try to decide whether the ad (1) gives straight information or whether it (2) is a virtue by association ad, (3) uses incomplete sentences, (4) offers an incomplete remedy, (5) is a fool's gold ad, or (6) tells you that food is love. Write the number of the ploy after each product type and see how often you are exposed to each.

Only by training yourself to interpret the advertisers' messages can you begin to make yourself immune to their effects.

When you work on cracking the advertisers' code, you are working on your own reeducation. It is a good idea to enlist the cooperation of your family. If you are the family food buyer, you can reeducate others so that they do not pressure you to bring into your home those troublesome excess foods. Even your preschool-age children can understand simple concepts like "good to eat" and "not good to eat" and they can begin to learn which messages tell less than the whole truth. Older children and spouses can join the game of "find the villain" as you all build your skills in wise consumerism.

2. Plan Your Attack

Frequency of exposure brings greater hazards of risk. The more frequently you enter the supermarket, the greater the possibility that you will make an unwise purchase. This is particularly true when you go into the market to buy only one or two items. You feel that you want to make the most of your trip or that you "should" buy several items, and therefore you pick up unnecessary items just to round out your purchases. Therefore, it is wise to *plan your shopping well in advance. Make as few shopping trips as possible, trying to go once each week or less.* If you have a tendency to run out of certain items, build up a supply. For example, if yours is a family which puts away two gallons of milk one week and three quarts the next, keep on hand a supply of powdered nonfat milk to draw upon in emergencies. If you have unexpected children staying for lunch and extra bread for sandwiches is needed, keep several loaves in the freezer so that you can avoid a shopping trip just to pick up a loaf of bread.

Prepare a list before you enter the store. It is a good idea to take advantage of weekly food specials. If you have the choice, shop at the market that has advertised specials on items which you need that week and try to buy only those things on your list. The three-for-a-dollar cookie specials and the day-old bakery items are problem merchandise for the market manager: let them be his problems and not yours—leave them alone! In order to plan your shopping in advance, *plan your menus at least a week in advance,* making certain that you estimate leftovers that will be available for lunches. If you go into the store without a list and look over everything on the shelves, there is a good chance that you will be hooked by the marketing and packaging specialist.

Shop only after you have eaten a satisfying meal and then only when you are feeling comfortable and rested. If you go into the store hungry, many food items will look good to you. If you feel hassled and harried, you will face the natural human inclination to buy a few treats as "pick-me-ups." Before you cross the threshold of the market, be sure your stomach is comfortably full and your spirits high.

3. On the Field of Battle

Store managers have become increasingly sophisticated. Music is now piped into climate-controlled emporiums. Display techniques have been developed in a way that offers products maximum eye appeal. Some larger markets even have snackbars. All of these creature comforts are designed to keep you in the store as long as possible because the longer you are "in house," the greater the possibility that you will snap up the bait. Therefore when you go into the store, *walk quickly, not slowly,* so that you minimize exposure to problem foods. *Walk only through the aisles that display foods that are on your list.* Again, the goal is to minimize your contact with problem foods. If possible, *shop with a friend* because this will help to sharpen your awareness of the products which you select. Take turns cross-examining each other: "Is this product really necessary?"

Remembering that the store manager displays products in a way that intensifies the likelihood of discretionary purchases, you can take the offensive and ask that staples be given prime shelf space. Ask that food bins near the checkout counter be replaced with magazine racks: you may as well thumb through the latest weeklies while you wait instead of trying to stifle your urge to buy things that you don't need. When you make progress with a store manager, tell your friends: help that manager make up in volume what might be lost through less impulse purchasing of unnecessaries.

IN A NUTSHELL

It is important for you to have in the house only those foods that you should eat. To help you restructure your buying to these and only these things, a multi-stage program has been suggested:

1. Build your resistance to commercials by watching as few as possible and by carefully analyzing the overt and covert messages of those that you do watch.
2. Cue other family members in so that they cut down their pressure on you to make unnecessary purchases.
3. Plan your shopping in advance, shop as seldom as possible, prepare your menus in advance and then develop a shopping list, and go into the store only when your resistance is high—when you're full and happy.
4. Finally, treat shopping like work instead of play: shop briskly, avoid contact with any foods that are not on your list, and try to shop with a friend with whom you can discuss the merits of problem purchases.

This program can go far toward helping you break the chain of problem eating at an early link by keeping problem foods where they belong: on the grocer's shelves instead of in your kitchen.

CHAPTER 6

Out of Sight, Out of Mind

SOME PEOPLE SEEM to eat too much too often. Others seem to eat just the right amount most of the time. How can we explain the difference? We could say that the people are different. However it would be closer to the truth to say that the people may be *slightly* different, but their major differences are to be found in their *eating environments*.

A number of factors help to clarify the picture of eating-urge control. The first is how hard one must work to find the food one eats. In one early study, newborn babies were given normal nipples on the first and third days of their lives and nipples with slightly smaller holes on their second day among us. Normal-weight babies worked a little harder and drew the same amount of milk on the second day as they did on the first and third. Overweight babies, however, drank 20 percent *less* on Day 2 than they did on Days 1 and 3.[1] Therefore, it should come as no surprise that overweight adults were later found to eat fewer nuts that required shelling and fewer chocolates that required unwrapping

65

while ease of access had little or no effect upon the
treats that the lean would eat.[2] Ease of access is therefore one important consideration.

The simple visibility of food is a second factor. When
food is out of sight, the overweight are less likely to
think about it than are the lean. When food is plainly in
view, on the other hand, the overweight will eat—
mealtime or not—and they will clean their plates of
every morsel. The lean are more likely to say "no thank
you" or leave a scrap or two.[3]

A third factor makes the picture even clearer. Research at Yale University has shown that the overweight
outperform the lean on tasks that require great attention
to detail—as long as there are no distractions. Add a
stimulus that can divert their attention, however, and
the performance of the overweight falls far below that
of the lean.[4] This tells us that the overweight attend
more closely to detail than do the lean, but perhaps
because of this their attention can be more easily distracted than can that of their normal-weight peers.

Using just these three factors, we can construct an environment that would make problem eating more likely
for the overweight although perhaps not for the lean:
make food easy to eat; put it in plain view; and provide
activities that are not totally absorbing so that the heavy
person's attention can be drawn to food.

We can also arrange an environment in which problem eating is *less* likely to occur, by providing foods that
take some effort to eat, by keeping these foods out of
view, and by providing strong non-food-related stimulation.

A Plan of Action

These important studies have given us the foundation
for a plan of action that can help to reduce the number
of times that eating is stimulated by carelessly managed
cues. If first you take the time to clean up your living environment, you will help yourself to *avoid* the tempta-

tions posed by food within easy reach. You will break the chain of eating urges early and preserve your second-strike capability. If, on the other hand, you leave your life space as it is, your only recourse will be to attempt to *escape* from temptation once it has arisen. The urge to eat will not only be stronger, but you will have no second chance. Therefore, great dividends can be gained through your willingness to act now to reduce the occurrence of eating crises.

Strategy 1. Clean House

Many temptations exist in every home and office. Any food that is on display or open for easy access is a trap. When your favorite bread is in a glass container, it is a temptation. The temptation is less when the container is opaque, and still less when the container is in a closed cupboard. Of course, buying breads that are not your favorites is an even better solution. If we reverse this sequence, we can list ways of managing the external environment so that problem eating is less likely to occur:

Don't buy foods that you have trouble resisting.
If you do buy these foods for others, keep them out of sight and reach.
Those foods which you can reach should be covered so that they offer as little temptation as possible.

Chapter 5 suggested ways to build control over the things that you buy. Now you can take steps to keep these foods out of reach and out of sight at home, at your office, and even when you go out to eat.
At home in your kitchen:

1. Put all foods in covered containers, whether they are on the counter, in the cupboard, or in the refrigerator;
2. Put favorite foods in the *least* obvious and most difficult-to-reach places;
3. Keep on the fronts of shelves only those foods whose temptation quotient is low.

At your *place of work,* have *no* food in your immedi-ate work area. Develop ways to handle food cues in the place that you eat your lunch. If the danger area is a cafeteria where you must pass a variety of tempting foods, plan to bring your lunch. If that is not practical, see if you can find someone who will buy your food for you so that you can skip the line entirely. And if that is not possible, try to find someone who will choose food for your tray while you choose food for his or hers.

In *restaurants,* you have the same goal: keep your contact with tempting foods to a minimum. You can do this by following the same food-cue hierarchy:

1. Select restaurants that serve the foods that you can and should eat;
2. Do not open the menu—order only what you know you should have;
3. Be the first to order, so that the foods chosen by others do not tempt you;
4. Request that condiments and rolls be moved to the far side of the table or be removed entirely, after others have had their fill.

Exotic restaurants may not serve the foods that you need: avoid these restaurants. Menus are written *in order to tempt you:* avoid reading them. If you must open a menu, look only at the salad and entrée section and avoid discovering that your passion foods are on the bill of fare. Even if the foods that you order are *not* on the menu, restaurants can often accommodate your wishes, so do not hesitate to ask. If you order your own food first, the choices of others will not tempt you. Finally, the removal of foods that are not part of your planned eating will help to curb your urge to eat them.

List the steps that you will follow in reducing contact with food cues in each of these environments:

1. _____
2. _____
3. _____

Strategy 2. Keep Busy

No matter how careful you are in eliminating eating cues from your environment, you must have food in the house. To keep from being drawn into the trap of eating the food that is unnecessary and unwanted, make sure that your attention is always occupied as constructively and enjoyably as possible. Food cues can distract you from your task, but a task that is interesting and challenging can also distract you from food!

Keep your mind busy with a range of absorbing activities. Crafts work well, and so do hobbies. If possible, have the supplies at hand and the work area already set up, so that you can pursue your activity at a moment's notice.

Often new books can be experienced as strangers. It takes effort to develop a "feel" for a new book so reading the first chapter can seem more like work than relaxation. Also, books have their own character and different books suit your needs when you experience different moods. At times when you feel bored or lonely —the kinds of times that usually trigger your urge to eat—it is useful to have at hand several books, the first chapters of which you have already read. That makes it easier to turn to reading as a source of stimulation. Having several books on hand will also make it more likely that you will have a novel, a book on current events, a humorous book, or any other kind of book that will meet your need when your urge to eat arises.

Phoning friends, doing chores—which could be anything from washing floors to balancing the checkbook—and listening to music or working on a craft project are other useful ways of attaining the goal of eating-urge control.

All of these strategies keep you in the situation in which the urge arises. If your eating urges occur at home, you might think of things to do outside the home during troublesome times. A visit to friends, a trip to the library, a full- or part-time job, or volunteer work can all help to divert you from the urge for food.

In the spaces below, list activities that you *now* enjoy that could be helpful in avoiding the urge to eat:

1. _____
2. _____
3. _____
4. _____

Now think of things that you do enjoy but have not done in some time, and other things that you would like to begin to do. List them in the following spaces:

1. _____
2. _____
3. _____
4. _____
5. _____

Look back over your lists and see which items you can do now with little or no preparation; star these. See which can be done with a small amount of preparation and put a plus by these. Next, make arrangements to get the activities under way. Start with those you have starred, move on to those that require a little more preparation, and finish with those for which the most preparation is necessary.

Specifically, your job here is:

PLAN TO USE AT LEAST ONE ACTIVITY
(WITH *TWO* OTHERS AS FALL-BACK PLANS)
DURING THE TIMES YOU NORMALLY FEEL
STRONG, TROUBLESOME URGES TO EAT.

To determine these times, look at the ratings that you gave your urge to eat in column 2 of the Self-Monitoring Chart on page 27.

What were the days when you were most likely to report more frequent non-hunger-related urges to eat?

At what hours did these urges arise?

What do you know about these particular days and these particular times that would allow you to plan activities that could subdue your urge to eat?

For example, Elaine found that her appetite was powerful in the late afternoon. Part of the problem was that she prepared dinner at this time and she tended to feel lonely by the end of the day. She decided to work on dinner right after lunch and use the time from 3:30 to 5:00 P.M. to do her gardening in good weather and her sewing when the weather was bad.

Bill found that he tended to start eating at dinner and to eat right through the evening. He realized that if he could break the grip of this habit of "needing" food, he would be home free all evening. He worked out an arrangement with his son Dan so that the two would work on their stamp collections together immediately after dinner. In short order, Bill's evening eating was brought under control and the D & B Stamp Plan Company was underway. These are the kinds of activities that you should arrange to help you cope with your high-stress times.

In a Nutshell

Researchers are gradually arriving at a description of those events in the environment that cue problem eating by the overweight. Easy access to food, food in full view, and vulnerability to distraction by food cues—all contribute to a buildup of eating urges. You can avoid giving in to temptation by following a two-stage plan of action. First, arrange your living environment so as to limit your access to problem foods. Second, build up your resistance to the food that must exist by providing for yourself a rich array of interesting activities that will draw your attention away from food.

CHAPTER 7

Making Eating
a Pure Experience

CYNTHIA HAS BEEN divorced for several years and she lives alone in a small apartment. She works hard at the office all day and comes home tired every evening. Because she puts out so much effort on the job, she likes to take it easy at home so dinner is usually broiled food eaten before the early-evening movie. When the film is over she clicks the TV off, does the dishes and a little straightening up, and spends an hour or two on work that she has brought home from the office. Then it is her custom to turn the TV back on to catch an interesting guest on a talk show or watch part of a late-night movie. Her problem is that she has grown from a size 10 to a size 16 in the past few years because her late-night televiewing is almost always coupled with an apple, then a slice of bread with a dab of peanut butter, and, when these have not hit the spot, a dish of ice cream with a handful of cookies.

What's happened to Cynthia? She has *trained* herself to turn to food whenever the TV tube comes to life. In this conditioned behavior she is not alone; millions of others put themselves to this same test every day. Let's look at just one of her fellow sufferers.

Ray is a member of a weight-conscious family. Everyone has a good breakfast and a well-planned, healthful dinner. There is no eating after dessert in the evening and everyone except Ray is trim and fit. What's Ray's problem? Well, he leads a very pressured day at work. He has a mountain of paperwork on all of his accounts and so he takes his coffee breaks at his desk and eats lunch there as well unless he has an appointment with a client (which almost always involves either lunch or coffee and a sweet roll). Over the months, Ray has learned that eating and working go together. As a result, he feels that his wits are dull and his concentration wanders unless he has a bite to eat. For his efforts, Ray has a full belly from nine to five, a paunch that makes him the black sheep of the family, and suits that come from the "Portly Shop" of the downtown department store.

Cynthia and Ray have learned to turn to food automatically when they do some of the important things in their lives. They are probably unaware of this self-programming, but they are painfully aware of its consequences. By being careless in allowing themselves to associate unnecessary eating with watching television and working, they have programmed into their lives habits that will be difficult to break.

We "program" ourselves to act in certain ways when we repeat several behaviors in the same sequence a few times over. This builds the habit strength of a chain of behaviors and in the future the occurrence of one response in the chain will make the next one very likely to occur. For example, Cynthia programmed herself to come home from work, put the groceries away, read the mail, put something in the broiler before hanging up her coat, splash some water on her face, and then wash the salad greens while the broiler does its work.

Ray arrives at his office at 9 and his first stop is at the coffee machine. He glances at the headlines of the newspaper as he sips his coffee and eats a Danish pastry as he opens his business mail and gets down to work. Like clockwork, one action follows upon the other and any step that is missed leads to an uncomfortable disruption of the routine.

As we move through our self-programmed paces, we also learn to associate certain stimuli with each action. Cynthia listens to the 6 o'clock radio news while she reads the mail: the news and mail go hand in glove for her. Ray opens the mail and eats his pastry: papers and pastries are a strong combination for him. After several weeks of these pairings, Cynthia's interest and comfort in reading the mail is "conditioned" to her hearing the newscast, and Ray's correspondence creates an urge to eat. This is the same conditioning that Pavlov discovered as a means of training his laboratory dogs to salivate when a bell was rung, after previously giving them food powder at the sounding of the bell. The only difference is that while Pavlov worked hard to condition his dogs, Cynthia and Ray simply *relaxed into their natural behavior chains to condition themselves in unintended ways.*

Why Should You Decondition Your Reactions?

Some conditioning is inevitable in everything we do. We cannot help but grow habituated to our routines and when we repeat behaviors in the same contexts, the contexts become cues to act. Much of this programming is harmless. For example, we dress ourselves in a fairly individual sequence—so what? We follow a common route in our drive or walk to work—that's okay too. We follow a routine when we settle down to relax in the evening and any change from that routine can interfere with our relaxation. That, too, is no problem. There is a problem, however, when the routines that we establish lead to an association between urges to eat and to activities that can and should be entirely free of food.

When we are careless and allow diverse activities to stimulate our appetite, we create for ourselves a continual pressure to suppress our appetite. It is easier to develop a negative reaction of this type than it is to bring it under control, but through effort we can learn to suppress the reaction entirely.

One advantage of *de*conditioning ourselves in this way is the freedom from an abiding preoccupation with food when we engage in diverse activities. Another advantage is that we can learn to perform these acts better and with more enjoyment if we can dissociate them from food. It has been pointed out that the overweight tend to be more distractable than those of normal weight. When appetite competes with another activity, the overweight experience difficulty in focusing their concentration. Therefore, eliminating food from other activities frees the individual to become involved in these tasks with total energy.

Separating eating from other activities can also help the reducer achieve a more accurate awareness of how much or how little he or she eats. Dr. Susan Wooley of the University of Cincinnati asked normal-weight and overweight subjects to recall the amount of food that they ate during an experimental meal. No group overestimated what they ate. Normal men underestimated by an average of 26 percent while overweight men underestimated by a full *44 percent*. Women did considerably better, with the normal-weight group testing out at an average of 7 percent off the mark as contrasted with 19 percent for the overweight group.[1] What this tells us is that under stimulus-controlled laboratory conditions, the overweight have a tendency to underestimate what they eat. When they are distracted from concentration on their food, it is reasonable to expect their accuracy to deteriorate even more.

Finally, when the overweight eat they experience what has been termed the "warm glow" syndrome. Their receptivity to many different stimuli is heightened and they predispose themselves to accept ideas that they might otherwise reject. For example, watching televi-

sion commercials while eating increases the likelihood
that the overweight will believe what they hear, while
watching the same commercials with no food at hand
denies the sponsor this unearned advantage.[2]

In summary, there are at least four advantages to be
gained from a serious effort at dissociating appetite
reactions from nonfood events. You can earn freedom
from a preoccupation with food at certain times, you
can gain more from the activities because you will not
be distracted by food, you can increase the likelihood
that you will be aware of what you eat, and you can
strengthen your critical faculties as you receive messages
aimed at influencing the way you think and feel.

Your Personal Deconditioning Program

To start your deconditioning program you must know
which situations are associated with your unguarded
eating. Typical cues are:

- Places,
- Activities, and/or
- People.

By looking at the times when you recorded a "—" in
columns 3 or 4 of your Urge to Eat Self-Monitoring
Chart (page 27), you can learn when you ate the wrong
foods or too much of the proper foods. Working back-
ward, you can then determine which places, activities,
and/or people tended to be present when these eating
problems arose.

Places

It is quite normal to think of food when you are in the
kitchen or dining room. If you have been careless about
the way in which you program your eating urges, you
must also have the urge to eat when you are in other

rooms of the house or other places in your life space. For example, if you keep a candy dish in the living room, walking into the living room can trigger the urge to eat a piece of candy. If you keep a dish of popcorn and nuts in the den, then merely stepping into the den can turn your attention to some nibbles. Therefore, you will have to make certain that you *keep food in the kitchen only* and that you *eat only in the kitchen or dining room.* This may mean removing the candy bars from the glove compartment of your car or the half-eaten packages of cookies that lie in wait in your lower right-hand desk drawer, in addition to purging the living room and den of their booby traps of treats.

Activities

Reading and watching television are the two most common activities which are associated with unguarded eating. Something as innocent as reading the morning newspaper while having breakfast can lead to the urge to eat when you read later in the day. Watching television while having dinner can program you to have that "empty" feeling when the television is turned on later in the evening. Some people eat when they work on craft projects, others when they engage in certain social activities like card playing and bowling. Whatever the activity, it is playing with fire for overeaters to condition themselves to feel the urge to eat at times of the day when by rights they should be urge-free.

People

Sometimes people are the cue for problem eating. Jane's sister used to bring homemade cakes and pies with every visit. Jane and Ellen could linger for hours over "coffee and . . ." When Ellen saw that Jane was putting on weight, she stopped bringing goodies. But Jane made certain that the table was spread, and in keeping up the tradition her bottom spread as well. For Jane, Ellen became a conditioned cue for the urge to eat. To keep the cost of sisterly love within bounds, Jane would have to work hard to reprogram her contacts with Ellen for both their sakes.

A Plan of Action

Working from these data you are now ready to get down to business. Make a pact with yourself to do three things:

1. Go through your home, car, and place of work on a shakedown search for any food. Remove all food to the kitchen.
2. Make a committment to do all of your eating only in specified places—
   a. In the kitchen, eat only when seated at your own place and then only when you use your own special placemat;
   b. In the dining room, also confine yourself to one chair and try to use a distinctive placemat;
   c. At work, eat only in the areas set aside for all workers to eat, or leave the building.
3. When you eat, make certain that eating is a pure experience by dissociating any and all activities other than socializing with family or friends.

Restricting all food to the kitchen will help you to overcome absentminded eating elsewhere. Eating at only one place in the kitchen or dining room will help you limit your eating urges to only these places.

Using a distinctive placemat will help you to gain even better stimulus control over the cues for eating urges because, when you have learned to allow *only the placemat* to trigger eating urges, you will be able to use your place at the table for other things as well. Finally, breaking the association between eating and other activities will allow you to enjoy both eating and the activities as uncontaminated, pure experiences.

In mounting this plan of attack you can anticipate two important difficulties. First, you must work toward *perfect consistency.* One or two slips will trigger the old expectancy mechanism all over again and you may spend weeks trying to regain your self-management controls. Therefore, once you make the decision to gain mastery over your urges to eat in this way, you must guard against a single error. With every slip you run the risk of telling your memory bank that the old rules are back in effect.

The other problem is faced by people who eat some or all of their meals alone. Singles or people whose spouses and families live and work on schedules different from theirs may find themselves in the habit of reading or watching television while eating. However strong the justification for pairing activities and eating, the effects are always the same: a constant need to fight a personal holding action to squelch the urge to eat. After trying to concentrate exclusively on eating for a week or two (once or twice is not enough!), try to choose as an eating activity something which you will do *at no other time of the day.* For example, if you tend not to read the newspaper you might pair it with eating. If you tend not to read magazines or books, they might be your mealtime company. If you generally ignore the radio, listening to local newscasts or to music might break the mealtime silence for you. It is best that you do nothing, but if you must do something try to make absolutely certain that it is not an activity which will cause eating-urge difficulties for you at other times of the day or night.

The simple steps suggested in this chapter can buy precious freedom for you—freedom from place-, activity-, and people-triggered urges to eat. By overcoming faulty conditioning in this way you can have the same degree of enjoyment of your life space that others have without feeling the need constantly to inhibit the desire to reach out for something to eat.

Use your Self-Monitoring Chart to keep track of your progress. In one of the unused sections of column 4,

draw a circle opposite the hours when you plan to take
particular care to work on your deconditioning program. Look over the chart at the start of each day to
remind yourself when special effort will be needed.
Then, as you go through the day, use these circled hours
to record a "+" if you have accomplished your objective and a "−" if greater effort is needed. Remember
that in this task *a perfect result is your goal*.

IN A NUTSHELL

In this chapter you have learned that there are routines in your behavior of which you may have been
unaware, and that many elements in this chain of behaviors are associated with stimuli in your immediate environment. You may have allowed certain places, activities, or people to stimulate your urge to eat, and merely
going to certain spots, doing certain things, or being
with certain people can bring your appetite to the fore.
These are conditioned associations between nonfood
stimuli and the urge to eat. To free yourself from these
unnecessary urges, you must work on deconditioning
yourself. You do this by making eating a pure experience, one that is not associated with any other event.
Make sure that all food is kept in your kitchen, that you
eat only in designated places, and that you engage in no
activity other than socializing with family, friends, or
business associates while you eat. Use your Self-Monitoring Chart to identify your danger signals and keep
track of your success.

CHAPTER 8

Eating Speed and Satisfaction

WHEN YOU ARE hungry, you will take frequent bites of your food and you will chew your food less thoroughly before you swallow. When you like the food, you will also take more frequent bites and chew less. When you are hungry, then, you are likely to eat as though you like the food you eat even though it might have little appeal at other times.[1] If you are overweight, you are also likely to take more bites, chew your food less, and take more food into your mouth per bite.[2]

The lean fill the between-bite time with many "thin eating behaviors." They put down their utensils between bites, they "toy" with their food, they wipe their mouths with their napkins, they leave scraps on their plates, and they rise from the table as soon as the meal has been eaten. The overweight, on the other hand, are all business. They eat quickly and efficiently, clean their plates completely, and yet linger at the table after the last morsel is gone as if hesitating to part from a beloved.[3]

The disadvantages of the rapid eating of the obese are obvious: they eat more than the lean per mealtime minute, they chew their food improperly so that it is less readily digested and absorbed, and in their haste they enjoy it less and so may be motivated to eat even more.

When obese and normal-weight volunteers were given exactly the same amounts of food and some were asked to eat quickly and others slowly, it was found that an hour later those who had eaten slowly were less hungry than those who had eaten at a more casual pace.[4]

Studies have shown that approximately twenty minutes are needed for the food that reaches the stomach lining to be broken down so that it can be absorbed into the bloodstream, for the absorption to take place, and for the blood to carry the message that nourishment has reached the stomach to the hunger centers in the brain. A surprisingly small amount of food is sufficient to trigger this "I've had my fill" signal, but a great deal of food can go down the hatch within that twenty minutes if the eating pace is fast.

Several explanations have been offered for this slow-eating/less-hunger relationship. When eating is slower, more chewing takes place and food is kept in the mouth longer. This means that the sensitive taste buds are stimulated longer and that the muscles in the jaw and tongue are more fully utilized. Both of these sensations can contribute to the feeling of satisfaction. (Children seem to know this. Given one cookie for dessert, most children learn to suck it slowly both to make it last longer and to increase satisfaction with the treat.) Chewing the food longer and extending the length of time that it is kept in the mouth can also help to increase its digestibility.

Chewing grinds food into smaller pieces which are better exposed to the digestive chemicals in the stomach and small intestine. Also, chemicals in the saliva help to start digestion before some foods reach the stomach and small intestine where digestion will be completed. Therefore, the chemical transformation of food from its solid state to a state in which it can pass into the blood system is expedited by slower chewing. The more efficient the digestion process becomes, the more quickly do chemical messages reach the brain to signal a stop to eating. Eating slowly, therefore, has the triple advantage of: (1) cutting down the amount which is eaten; (2) making the food that is consumed more digestible; and (3) increasing the feeling of satisfaction that follows the consumption of moderate amounts of food.

What Can Be Done?

Are you likely to be the first to finish a meal? Does the serving of food cause you to stop talking and start eating while others continue to participate in conversation? Do you tend to hold onto your fork or spoon from the first bite until the last bite of food has been eaten? Do you tend to put more food into your mouth before you have swallowed the food which was already there?

Whether or not you think about eating all day long, are you relatively unaware of the taste, smell, and texture of the food that you eat while you are eating it? Can you recall whether you can feel the seeds in tomatoes with your tongue? Whether eggs have a distinctive aroma? Or whether roast beef is sweeter or saltier than steak? And do you find yourself still thinking about food when you have finished what you know to be an adequate meal? These are the signs of *someone who must learn again how to eat*—strange as that may seem.

What you must learn to do is to s-l-o-w d-o-w-n the rate at which you eat. To do this, you will have to select one or more of the following steps to follow *at your main meal:*

1. When you sit down at the table with others, keep your utensils on the table for the first two minutes of the meal as you think quietly to yourself about how you will work on slowing down the rate of your eating.

FIGURE 8.1

Self-Monitoring Chart for Rate of Eating

	How many minutes did you spend eating your main meal?			Did you take these steps?				After eating your normal meal, how did you feel?	
	Time start?	Time stop?	Total time?	2-min. wait?	Cut food?	Put fork down?	Sense taste, texture, smell?	Less satisfied than normal?	More satisfied than normal?
Monday									

Wednesday ———

Thursday ———

Friday ———

Saturday ———

Sunday ———

2. Before you start to eat, cut the food on your plate into small bite-sized portions.

3. Pick up your fork and put one portion in your mouth, putting the fork down as soon as it is empty.

4. Chew the food carefully and thoughtfully. Feel the texture of the food with your tongue as it is ground into smaller morsels by your teeth. Try to sense its saltiness or sweetness, its bitterness or its sourness. Concentrate on smelling its aroma. Focus your attention upon the experience of eating so that you can capture its full enjoyment.

5. When the food has been swallowed, join in the conversation before picking up your fork for another bite which will again become the focus of your attention.

6. Finally, make certain that you are the last person to start to eat each new course as it is served. You will do this in order to extend to the maximum possible the time which you spend eating your meal.

Steps one, five, and six will help to extend the length of time that you spend eating. Step one is particularly important because it has been observed that eating rate during the first five minutes of the meal sets the rate of eating throughout the meal.[5]

Steps two and three will help you to take smaller bites and to keep only a moderate amount of food in your mouth at any one time.

Step four will help you savor the food that you are eating, and this will ultimately help you to enjoy your eating more. Strange as it may seem, while many overweight people spend their lives thinking about food, they often eat it so fast that they hardly ever fully experience it.

Which of the steps will you choose to follow? As with all of the other recommendations in this book, it is important to be able to keep track of your progress. A special self-monitoring chart (see Figure 8.1) should be used for following your progress with this particular series of steps.

Bring this chart to the table with you for your main meal for seven consecutive days. Check your start and stop times. Become aware of your effort to develop the "thin eating behaviors": pause before starting, cut food carefully, set your utensils down between mouthfuls, and concentrate on the taste, texture, and smell of the food that you are chewing slowly. Then, when the meal is done, rate your satisfaction with your new eating style. You should find that satisfaction mounts as your eating rate declines.

IN A NUTSHELL

The obese and the lean eat at very different rates. The obese eat normally in the same way that the lean eat when they are very hungry and are eating a favorite food—that is, with little time between bites, larger bites, and little time to chew. This "fat" eating pattern leads to consumption of a large amount of food before satiety is experienced, to swallowing food in relatively un-digestible form, and to a diminished sense of satisfaction after the meal has ended. The result is that the obese are ready to eat sooner after a meal than the lean. To correct this situation, it is recommended that the overweight adopt a program of six steps toward the development of a "lean eating pattern." Included among these steps are recommendations that you wait two minutes before eating while you plan your slower eating pace, that you place your utensils on the table between mouthfuls, and that you chew your food very slowly, concentrating on its taste, smell, and texture.

CHAPTER 9

Timing Your Urge to Eat

Invisible rhythms underlie most of what we assume to be constant in ourselves and the world around us. Life is in continual flux, but the change is not chaotic. The rhythmic nature of earth life is, perhaps, its most usual yet overlooked property. Though we can neither see nor feel them, we are nevertheless surrounded by rhythms.[1]

DO YOU LIKE to eat a hearty breakfast or does food taste like sawdust in your mouth before midday? If you have a "taste for food" one morning, you are almost sure to have it the next; and if you escape breakfast one day, food will taste no better at dawn the next. This is because your taste sensation follows a circadian or 24-hour cycle along with nearly all of your important bodily functions.[2] Indeed, in you and in all life around you, rhythms measure and control the pace of life.

Rhythm implies time and time is a crucial dimension

in eating control. You may not be able to change the diurnal nature of your taste sensation, but you can alter the time each day that it is strong or weak. People who have been closed off from all cues of natural day or night nevertheless follow almost perfect sleep-wake cycles in a 24-hour pattern. Others whose fluid intake varies greatly from one day to the next produce urine with remarkable regularity. Just as you could, with difficulty, shift the time of your taste for food by training yourself to start your circadian rhythm in motion at different times of day, so, too, can you train yourself to experience the urge to eat at different times of day.

Research done at Columbia University in the mid-1960s first alerted weight-control experts to a very important fact: overweight people tend to feel the urge to eat when *they think* their mealtimes have arrived.[3] Student volunteers were seen in an experimental room in which the time shown on the clock was artificially manipulated. For some subjects the clock time was regulated to pass much more slowly than real time, while for others the time shown on the clock was speeded up considerably. During the experiment, subjects were given the opportunity to eat crackers, and the number eaten was carefully observed by the research team. It was found that normal-weight people were not influenced by manipulated time: they ate the same number of crackers whether the time was apparently passing quickly or slowly. Overweight people, on the other hand, seemed to be very much influenced by apparent time. They ate significantly *fewer* crackers when they thought that their normal dinner hour had *not yet arrived* and they ate significantly *more* crackers when they believed that their dinner hour had *already passed*. Overweight people, unlike those of normal weight, appeared to be more influenced by the clock than the natural time of day.

Elsewhere it has been shown that when overweight people were denied access to any external cues about time, they were much more varied in their estimates of lapsed time than were normal-weight subjects who seemed to be less dependent upon external time cues.[4]

On the basis of the above facts, there is good reason to believe that *scheduled* eating can have an important *positive impact* upon the urge to eat experienced by overweight people.

Patterns of Eating

People eat on some very different schedules.[5] In general, three different patterns have been demonstrated. In one, certain quantities of food are eaten at certain times every day. When this plan is followed for several weeks, thoughts of eating are confined to the scheduled times. If the eating times coincide with the best conditions for controlling the amount and selection of food for that individual, this kind of eating pattern is constructive and well adapted to the individual's needs.

A second pattern is found among those who decide to "diet" every day. This decision usually means delaying any eating as long as possible, sometimes throughout the entire day, and eating at will during the evening. Hunger is rarely experienced during the daylight hours but it is a constant companion during the evening.

A third pattern is one in which eating is scheduled but the times selected are not those designed to produce the best self-control. Breakfast is likely to be skipped, as is lunch. Dinner is generally a full meal with snacks planned for several times during the evening. Eating during the evening is often a problem because most people are less occupied then as opposed to during the day and therefore they have fewer opportunities to distract themselves from food thoughts once the thoughts have begun. The problem with this third eating schedule is that food is not available when eating is most controllable and is available when eating is most likely to resist control.

A Plan of Action

In order to achieve freedom from obsessive preoccupation with food, you must set up a systematic program whereby you eat at only specified hours. This will condition your body to expect food at certain times and not at others. Our bodies are dominated by patterns of consistency, despite their vast complexity. Therefore, the achievement of urge-free times during the day requires a highly consistent restraining effort. Two things are necessary:

> FIRST YOU MUST DECIDE WHEN
> YOU WOULD LIKE TO EAT EVERY DAY.
> THEN YOU MUST FOLLOW THIS SCHEDULE
> FOR SEVERAL CONSECUTIVE WEEKS.

How often should you eat? This is a question that has interested health professionals for many years. No one knows what our natural eating rhythm might be because throughout human history we have sacrificed our natural tendencies to cultural conventions.[6] Meat-eating animals tend to gorge themselves when they make a kill while grass-eating animals tend to take in small amounts of food constantly. Because man is both meat and vegetable eating, our natural pattern would probably be a cross between the gorging of the meat eaters and the nibbling of the grass eaters.

Different eating patterns can have some impact upon health. Research has shown that people who have fewer than three meals each day tend to have slightly higher cholesterol and triglyceride levels and lower glucose tolerance levels.[7] Both of these are problems for the overweight. Other studies have shown that those who eat fewer than three meals per day also have a slightly greater chance of experiencing certain kinds of heart disease.[8] Eating three meals per day and avoiding the urge to skip breakfast and lunch can therefore bring with it some important health advantages. Although other studies have shown that it may not have a *necessary* impact upon the management of weight,[9] eating three meals per day can also help to reduce that "psychological caloric deficit" which leads many people to feel that they owe themselves extra calories because they passed up food at normal mealtime hours.

For these reasons, it is important that you plan to have *three square meals per day.* At the start, you should plan to have these three meals *at the most conventional times of day,* starting with an early-morning breakfast. Even though you may not like the taste of food in the early morning, you can condition yourself to shift the inner cycle of your food interest and in doing so you can bring your eating under the normal conditions that will help you to limit both what and how much you eat. You may not like food at the start; if so, you can begin with a light breakfast and gradually build up. Eventually, consistency will help you to change what you may have regarded as an irreversible dislike of food at various times of day.

You may also plan to have snacks when you feel that they are important. Snacks must be within the range of foods and within the portions that are permitted by the food plan that you are following. When snacks are chosen, they must be taken with the same care that meals are eaten: eat them in the proper place, control access to seconds, and do nothing else while eating. You must also *schedule the exact time of your snacks just as carefully as you schedule your meals.*

You may vary the scheduled times of your meals or snacks by up to twenty minutes or so from day to day, *but greater variations defeat the purpose of the reconditioning program* that you have chosen to follow. Therefore, you will have to be prepared to discipline yourself on weekends as well as on weekdays, having breakfast, lunch, dinner, and any planned snacks at roughly the same time every day.

By now you may be wondering whether it is worth the bother to get up for breakfast at the same time on weekends as on work days, or to play havoc with your social schedule by insisting upon dinner at the same time throughout the week. Only *you* can decide. If freedom from persistent urges to eat is important to you, the effort necessary to restrain yourself to think of food *only at the times that you choose* will be a small price to pay.

Once you have reconditioned yourself to think of food at certain times only, you can go back to a more natural flexibility. As you will learn when you make this deconditioning effort, this urge-to-eat pattern develops a definite strength and resilience that can become strong enough to withstand a reasonable amount of variability.

If you are willing to make the effort, circle the hours of your planned three meals and snacks, if you choose them, on the Urge to Eat Self-Monitoring Chart and then record your success in eating at these times only.

As the weeks progress, data recorded on the chart will also give you a very good way to evaluate your success. You should find that you record fewer incidents in column 2 when your appetite is strong between scheduled meal hours. Demonstrating changes in your appetite in this way will help you to see just how well you are succeeding in this important self-restraining effort.

In a Nutshell

Many of your most important biological processes follow a 24-hour cycle. While you cannot control the recurrence of the cycle, you can control the time that it begins and ends. This chapter has suggested that you choose times to eat and that you eat at these times only. After a matter of weeks you should find that your thoughts turn to food at preplanned hours only.

CHAPTER 10

Managing Appetite by Day and by Night

MAN IS ONE of the few species that enjoys the "privilege" of eating when not hungry and drinking when not thirsty.[1] This privilege is one of the banes of our existence because it lies at the root of our chronic overeating and overweight.

In theory, we should be hungry when our bodies have used up their available supply of nutrients and we should feel no hunger when our nutrient supply is adequate. In practice, however, even if our body's needs have been met, we feel "hungry" when:

1. We have not had a sufficient range of tastes and food textures to satisfy our need for these experiences;
2. We believe that we have not had enough to eat;
3. We are in contact with tempting foods; or
4. We turn to food to meet psychological needs.

At these times, our feeling is not hunger, but appetite, a major link in the problem eating chain.

Variety in Your Diet

During World War II, GIs ate tens of millions of cartons of K rations. This bland, dehydrated, and canned food provided all of their minimum daily nutrient requirements. But many soldiers complained that they could survive on these rations much longer than they cared to live.[2] Their hunger was appeased but their appetites remained unsatisfied. The reaction of these GIs demonstrated that "full" and "satisfied" are very different experiences.[3]

Recent lab studies have come to the same conclusion. Volunteers were allowed to drink their fill of a liquid diet that contained all of the necessary nutrients and calories, and yet the urge to eat was almost unabated: the subjects drank no more than they needed, but they were preoccupied with eating and longed for solid food.[4]

This has a very important implication for you.

IN ORDER TO LIMIT ONE SOURCE OF
"HUNGER" DURING OR BETWEEN MEALS,
MAKE CERTAIN THAT YOU EAT A VARIETY
OF FOODS WITH DIFFERENT APPEARANCES,
TASTES, AND TEXTURES.

Do not choose a diet in which the same foods turn up on your plate time and time again. You must *plan for variety: it will not happen by itself.* Vary the colors, tastes, and smells of your preselected foods so that every meal includes variety and so that few foods are repeated at less than three- or four-day intervals.

Be certain that you have a range of foods that require biting and chewing at no less than two of your three daily meals.

The failure to exercise the muscles of your mouth and tongue can contribute to your feeling of not having had enough to eat.

Satiety Is in the Eye of the Beholder

The liquid diet studies have taught us other lessons as
well. Lean and obese volunteers in these studies were
given liquids with different caloric densities: sometimes
the fluids looked rich, sometimes thin; regardless of
their appearance, the liquids sometimes had high caloric
value, sometimes low. The volunteers therefore did not
know whether they were getting liquid that was rich or
poor in calories. We have learned from these studies
that:

1. Both the lean and the obese misjudged the caloric density of their meals, often thinking that high was low and
   that low was high;
2. Over time, both groups learned to adjust the caloric
   value of their intake to a constant level, requiring them
   to drink more on some days, less on others; and
3. When the volume of the drink was high, even if the
   caloric density was low, the volunteers reported feeling
   more satisfied than when the drink volume was low but
   the caloric value was high.[5]

In short, whether fat or thin, we tend to feel the urge
to eat until we *think* that we have had enough to eat: actually having enough to eat is not enough to do the
trick.

You can put these important observations to work for
you at mealtimes by taking three very useful steps:

1. Plan to begin your noon *and* evening meals with a
   generous salad using vegetables that are permitted in
   comparatively large quantity according to the food plan
   you are following. This will help to increase the bulk of
   your meal.
2. Eat your meal on a 7-inch salad plate so that it appears
   to be larger in quantity.
3. Serve all foods in carefully measured portions and take
   second helpings only of those foods which are unlimited
   in the food plan you are following. That way you will
   know exactly when you have had your fill. To make this

easier, serve "hotel" rather than "boardinghouse" style, with serving platters kept *off* the table.

By chewing vigorously at the start of your noon and evening meals, you are likely to feel satisfied sooner because your biting and chewing needs have been at least partially satisfied. If you eat your meal on a 7-inch salad plate rather than a 9-inch dinner plate, you increase the apparent size of your portion. The larger it looks, the more likely you are to feel satisfied. And by serving yourself your full portion at the start of the meal and not going back for seconds, you will learn to be satisfied with one measured helping.

Managing Nighttime Eating

Two out of three reducers interviewed by one eminent researcher reported that they did most of their eating at night.[6] Fifty percent of those who participated in a study conducted among members of Weight Watchers classes at the beginning of their weight-loss efforts reported that they, too, ate and ate and ate after the sun went down.

Night eaters have different food preferences. Some eat bread, others sweets. And they eat at different times. Some eat heavily between dinner and bedtime. Others rise after falling asleep and find their way to the kitchen. Some try valiantly to control their nocturnal eating. Others simply relax and enjoy it. But all have two things in common. First, they are nearly always breakfast avoiders and lunchtime nibblers. Their first hearty meal is very likely to be dinner. Second, they consistently report that early in the day they experience a strong aversion to the very foods which they find so irresistible at night.

Their skipping of meals early in the day paves the way for their nighttime eating. First, it creates hunger. These people are not necessarily physically hungry; their bodies have more than an adequate supply of energy in the form of convertible fat. But they have not had an opportunity to stimulate their taste buds, to exercise their chewing muscles, and to experience the sensation of food entering their stomachs. These are important physical sensations, the absence of which can be very disquieting.

The omission of meals early in the day also creates a "psychological caloric debt." Night eaters often feel that because they have been so "good" during the day, they owe themselves an extra treat at day's end. They may sometimes forget that they ate a particular food during the day, but their debit bookkeeping abilities are unsurpassed and they virtually never forget snacks which they have passed by.[7]

While there is a diabolical quality to their efforts to make up for lost treats, nighttime eaters may actually have a biological reason for enjoying their food more at night than during the day. The biorhythmic hormonal cycles mentioned in Chapter 9 affect the acuity of all of our senses at different times during each 24-hour period. For example, we may be bothered by the sounds of children's play at night but hardly notice it during the day. We may find bright lights glaring at night but walk about without sunglasses at high noon. We may feel sexually aroused in the evening by a person whom we hardly noticed during the day. We may also find the taste of some foods irresistible in the evening although we found them distasteful throughout the day.

Each of these sensory reactions could be influenced by secretions from various endocrine glands which shield us from strong reactions at some times of the day and intensify our reactions at others. Whatever the mechanism, there does appear to be good reason for believing that many foods taste better, at least to some people, after the sun goes down.[8]

In addition to hunger and heightened taste sensitivity, there is a third factor that makes nighttime eating a particular problem. There are usually fewer social and situational controls at night, controls that would help to put the brakes on problem eating. Nighttime eaters often eat alone because other members of their family are either occupied or asleep. They often feel let down at the prospect of long nighttime hours with little stimulation. In the morning, for example, they may anticipate the day's work and not feel the need to turn to food as a diversion. They may also find that they are particularly bored and lonely at night when there are fewer activities that can compete with food for their attention.

Whatever the personal combination of events, the end result is usually the same: the after-dark eater is likely to go beyond the limits of prudent eating. Careful steps must be taken to prevent this eating from getting out of hand.

Eating Before Bedtime

As a first step, all nighttime eaters must make it a hard and fast rule to *eat three full, planned meals at the appropriate times every day.* This rule must be followed *even if eating has occurred the night before.* Unfortunately, when people do eat at night, they attempt to "pay back" the extra calories the following day by skipping breakfast and possibly lunch as well. In so doing, they pass up nutritionally sound foods that could be eaten at times when control is strong. They then arrive at home in the evening overhungry and with weakened resolve. This sets the stage for a second night of eating foods with the lowest nutritional value.

When three meals have been eaten, the continuing urge to eat before bedtime must be considered *mood-motivated eating.* In other words, appetite after dark (it cannot be hunger if the three meals have been eaten) is *not* a sign that food is needed but a *signal* that you are bored, unhappy, angry, or anxious. As you will learn in Chapter 11, the remedy for boredom is to find a stimulating alternative to eating. For unhappiness, the remedy is to seek constructive help from others. For anger, the remedy is assertion to correct a difficult situation. And meditation or other relaxation techniques are a more constructive response to anxiety than eating.

In addition to following one of the mood-management programs, it is also helpful to think of the evening as a series of thirty-minute, fifteen-minute, or even five-minute intervals that you believe you can successfully manage. Your goal then is to plan an activity that will get you through each time interval. When you plan activities in these small time units, you are always close to your next success—living through several more minutes without resorting to eating.

Use a chart like that in Figure 10.1. Write out your plan so that it is more concrete and specific. Whenever you write "No" on your chart, it is time for you to:

1. Analyze what has happened;
2. Plan a new activity for the next unit of time;
3. And go on with this next step *without dwelling* on your earlier mistake.

In other words, a slip-up in your behavior *is not an indication that you are a failure:* it merely means that the plan you followed earlier was not equal to the task at hand. With more careful planning you should achieve greater success. In addition, the more times that you prove to yourself that you are controlling nighttime eating, the less you will be preoccupied with that danger in the future. You are building confidence for future nights.

Waking Up to Eat After Falling Asleep

People who get up in the night to eat have a tendency to hide their eating from those with whom they live. Eating when they are still drowsy after having awakened helps them further hide their eating from themselves. Many state that they cannot recall whether, if, and how

FIGURE 10.1

Breaking Long Evenings into Small Challenges

Time		What I will do	Did I do it?		Did I succeed in controlling my eating?	
(Choose the interval which works best for you)		(Naturally, you should choose activities which interest you)	*Yes*	*No*	*Yes*	*No*
From	To					
7:00	7:30	Watch evening news	Yes		Yes	
7:30	8:00	Do ironing, wash dishes, fix lunch for tomorrow	Yes		Yes	
8:00	8:30	Call Alice, Tom	Yes		Yes	
8:30	9:00	Complete math lesson plan	Yes		Yes	
9:00	9:30	Read novel	Yes		Yes	
9:30	10:00	Continue reading	Yes		Yes	
10:00	10:30	Shower, choose clothes for tomorrow	Yes		Yes	
10:30	11:00	Catch up on correspondence	Yes		Yes	
11:00		To sleep				

much they ate. Unfortunately, however, it is all too obvious when a number of these late-night bouts have been fought and lost.

A five-step plan has proven to be highly effective in breaking the pattern of middle-of-the-night eating.

1. Early in the evening, prepare a small snack of an acceptable and nonpreferred food, like celery, lettuce, cauliflower, or other vegetable that you can bite and chew with no dip or dressing. Make sure that the food that you choose is not one of your favorite treats. In addition, the food should be low in caloric value and it should be a food that will not tax your resistance.

2. Drink no fluids for the six or seven hours before you retire, even if this means nothing to drink from as early as 4 P.M. on. The reason for this is that most middle-of-the-night eaters claim that their sleep is broken by the urge to void, with thoughts of eating coming *after* they have awakened for another reason.

3. Whether or not you wake up because you must go to the bathroom, pause a moment and remind yourself of the next step.

4. This step requires that you return to bed for a ten-minute wait. Practice meditation or another relaxation exercise (see page 136). If you fall asleep, good. If you do not fall asleep and find that your thoughts still turn to food, then you may go to the kitchen.

5. When you get to the kitchen, turn on the bright lights. Take the snack that you have prepared for yourself to the kitchen or dining room table. Use your own placemat and sit in your usual place. Eat the food slowly and concentrate on its taste and texture.

Each of these steps is important because each helps you to be aware of your eating, an awareness that can do much to build your control. Each step offers a means of breaking another link in the appetite chain. You have made it less likely that you will wake up. If you do awaken, you will try a primary line of defense by delaying your eating. If you still feel the urge to eat, that eating will be as much as possible under your conscious control. Finally, you will have demonstrated to yourself

FIGURE 10.2

Scorecard for Managing Nighttime Eating

	Mon.	Tues.	Wed.	Thurs.	Fri.	Sat.	Sun.
Prepared an acceptable snack							
Remembered to limit fluids before bedtime							
Did wake up to go to bathroom							
Did wait 10 minutes							
Did turn on kitchen lights, take prepared snack, and eat at my place at the table							
Did manage to eat only my prepared snack							

that you can have mastery over your eating impulses even when you are the weakest and your impulses the strongest.

If eating during the night is a problem for you, use the chart in Figure 10.2 to keep a record of your efforts and the results. You may have to experiment a bit with your own reactions in order to find the proper combination of techniques that is best for you.

IN A NUTSHELL

Management of daytime eating begins with variety in your diet. Research has shown that you must have taste and texture variety if you are to feel satisfied with what you eat. Because you are more likely to feel satisfied with your meals if you "think" you have had enough, you will also help to reduce your appetite for unnecessary food by making your portions appear larger and by making second helpings a thing of the past.

Night eating, before or after bedtime, is one of the most insidious habits faced by overeaters. Like a brush fire in a windstorm, once it begins there is much to keep it going and little to stop its spread. The most prudent approach to controlling night eating is to adopt a preventive approach. To control before-bedtime night eating, eat three meals daily and then plan short-duration activities that occupy your attention elsewhere. For after-bedtime eating, minimize the likelihood that you will awaken after retiring, but be prepared with an acceptable, nonpreferred snack and a definite plan of action that will make you very much aware of everything you do.

CHAPTER 11

Controlling the Moods Behind Your Urge to Eat

PEOPLE'S FANCIES TURN to food when their emotions are aroused. GIs in World War II who crouched in their foxholes would reach into their rucksacks for a bite to eat. After the death of a loved one, mourners eat to help themselves cope with their loss. And fans in the stands of closely contested (but not one-sided) ballgames eat junk food by the pound. Throughout recorded history, emotions and food have been closely linked.

Although the data are by no means clear-cut on this important topic, most researchers believe that the over-weight tend to be more emotional than the lean, and are also more likely to turn to food at times of stress.[2]

Irrespective of who does it more, the obese and the lean can and often do fall victim to the same vicious cycle:

1. Something in the environment triggers a strong emotion;
2. The person turns to a small amount of food;

3. The food is no match for the emotions; but
4. The eating itself sets off a secondary and often equally strong guilt reaction;
5. This guilt reaction leads to further eating or larger quantities of food.

Once this cycle begins, the more you eat the worse you feel; the worse you feel the more you eat—there's no way out until you're exhausted or the cupboard is bare.

Two emotions that often start this cycle are anxiety and depression. Anxiety is a feeling of tension that carries with it worry, inattention, distractibility, forgetfulness, heart palpitations, pounding pulse, sweating, headache, stomach distress, and many other symptoms. Everyone experiences some anxiety, and each of us probably experiences at least mild anxiety almost every week. Anxiety is a dread of some feared experience, but the threat that elicits anxiety is vague and amorphous, (as compared to fear, where the threat is, specific and focused). Because the threat in anxiety is not specific, the individual does not have a clear direction in which to respond. Nevertheless, the body becomes aroused as if to make a response. In effect, the individual is all geared up to take action, but no action is available. The result is a kind of cognitive, physiological, and behavioral wheel-spinning in which all systems are highly active and utterly unproductive.

While anxiety is a fear of some unknown future event, depression is a reaction to unhappy past events. Depression is a feeling of despair, bringing with it pessimistic, melancholic, and self-depreciating thoughts and a slowness of speech, movement, and activity. Sometimes depression is brought on by the loss of an important relationship or opportunity, which leads to the withdrawal of support for familiar patterns of behavior.

For example, if you are accustomed to having morning coffee with a friendly neighbor and that neighbor moves away, you may undergo a midmorning depression without being aware of it, simply because your routine has been disrupted.

At other times depression is the result of constant attacks—real or imagined—against which the individual feels defenseless. And sometimes depression is an outgrowth of past failures that make the prospect of future success seem all but nonexistent.

The common thread in both anxiety and depression is the frustration that the individual experiences whenever an effort is made to find a solution to a problem. For the anxious person, everything is tried but nothing works because the threat has a thousand ever-changing faces. For the depressed person, nothing is tried because nothing can work, as "proven" by countless failures in the past.

Boredom and anger are two other emotions that commonly trigger problem eating. Boredom is the result of living or working in an understimulating environment. In such environments our attention drifts aimlessly and painfully. Physical and psychological illness can result if we live for long in an environment that lacks the stimulation that we need to feed our tireless brains. When boredom becomes acute, we can panic. Because the overweight tend to be more sensitive to their environments (see Chapter 6), boredom may affect their behavior more quickly than that of the lean.

While boredom arises when nothing happens in the environment, anger is provoked by something that either did happen or was believed to have happened. Injury, insult, or mistreatment can cause the person to strike out. Sometimes direct action is possible and the injured party will retaliate against the provoker. But at other times direct action is not possible, and aggression will be directed against innocent bystanders (who are guilty by association), or against oneself. That overweight children sometimes learn to cram food into their mouths as a means of expressing anger against their parents is an illustration of self-directed anger. Unfortunately, many learn to carry this same frustration and self-defeating response into adulthood.

Stress is the fifth reaction that is frequently associated with overeating. Properly speaking, it is more than a mood, but it acts in many of the same ways, and it is most readily controlled through use of any of a number of mood-management techniques.

We tend to think of stress as a negative experience, when in fact it has some very important positive implications. On the positive side, stress is the response that triggers our adaptive energies when an active reaction is demanded. For example, without a stress response we might not jump out of the path of an onrushing car or quickly find the right words to say to a teenager who has decided to leave home in response to a family conflict. These stress reactions are adaptive as long as we can make responses that we believe have some reasonable chance of being effective. However, when a response is necessary and we have none that seem to work, inner pressure builds to the point where we experience negative stress in our bodies and in our emotions. The manifestations of this reaction are universal; we all have them to some degree almost every day of our lives. Physiologically we sense a tightness in our stomachs, or experience headaches, blurred vision, flushing, fatigue, changes in body chemistry, and more. Psychologically we may find our emotional thresholds lower, so that we respond too strongly too soon, in addition to feeling frustrated and overwhelmed. When overstressed, we frequently become prone to impulsive, unwise decisions, one of which can be to overeat.

Overeating is a high-probability response to all five of these emotional experiences. Why? It does not help the situation in any way; instead, it tends to make matters worse because of the guilt it carries with it. Its only real function seems to be distraction, because to the extent that we devote our thoughts to food we free ourselves from thinking about the real problems. In other words, through what may be lifelong habits, we often seek in the pantry solutions to our problems, the result being that we end up feeling worse than we felt at the beginning.

In summary, anxiety, depression, boredom, anger, and stress are the five emotions that can trigger impulsive eating. All five emotions have both thought and behavioral components that can be summarized as follows:

	Thought Component	Behavioral Component
Anxiety	Something terrible is going to happen.	Fast and furious attempts to find something—anything—that will defend one against the danger.
Depression	I have made errors in the past and am doomed to make the same mistakes again and again.	Inactivity because nothing helps.
Boredom	I have interests and needs, but the environment does not support either.	Alternation between a frantic search for stimulation and resigned inaction.
Anger	My rights have been carelessly or intentionally violated.	Counter-aggression against the provoker when possible, against oneself at other times.
Stress	I am helpless. Nothing I can do will make things better.	Paralysis—doing nothing—or lunging out in various poorly planned efforts.

As you can see, each of the emotions is connected with a belief system that may be accurate, but is usually incorrect; and all have behavioral components which frequently lead to unproductive actions that only serve to compound the problem.

A Critical Choice

When one of these moods descends, three alternatives are open to you:

1. You can do nothing, acquiesce, and suffer through.
2. You can take steps to change the offending situation.
3. You can try to contain the emotion.

Acquiesence means blindly accepting suffering that is as painful as it is unnecessary. Changing the situation not only permits the termination of your pain, but it creates the opportunity for pleasure. Containing the emotion allows the situation to exist as a source of stress, but focuses your attention on means of reducing the pain. A simple analogy may make the choice clear. If you have a headache that you know to be the result of stress, you can do one of the following: you can "tough it out" and simply hope for the pain to come to a prompt and merciful end; you can do all that is in your power to end the tension-causing stress; or you can continue to struggle in a stressful situation but take aspirin to curb your pain. The first option exposes you to useless suffering. The second holds the promise of long-term cure. And the third brings immediate relief. You would be wise to choose the latter two.

Our choice of one of these alternatives is likely to be governed by the way we label the situations in which we find ourselves. For example, as I rushed to meet the deadline for submitting this manuscript to the publisher, one of my sons asked for a ride to a debate tournament some eight miles away. My initial automatic reaction was one of stress tinged with anger as I asked myself: "How am I going to finish this work on schedule if my kids persist in springing time-consuming surprises on me at the last minute?" The labels that I put on the situation were negative, i.e., "too much to do in too little time," and "I'm a victim of my son's lack of consideration." Both labels encouraged further negative emotions, and neither label could lead to constructive action.

I did have other choices, however. For example, I could have labeled the request as an opportunity to do something for my son that would show him I consider his wishes to be on a par with my own. I could also have labeled it as an opportunity to do some limit-setting that would allow each of us to consider the other's desires more effectively in the future. Negative labels would not have triggered constructive action, while positive labels would have opened the door to corrective action.

Armed with positive labels, I might have acquiesed and simply taken my son to the debate, planning to stay up a few hours later to compensate for lost time. I could also have used this one last pressure to call the publisher to negotiate a more realistic deadline, or I could have called other parents and attempted to negotiate an exchange of chauffeuring services that would have allowed me to finish my work as planned. Finally, I could have stood my ground but gone for a ten-minute jog to work off my tension before settling down again to work.

Setting Your Sights

When troublesome emotions occur, it is always better to do something than to do nothing. This means that you must either try to change the situation or the emotions generated by the events. It also means that there is a choice to be made, and you must have a dependable means of making the correct decision. With no clear goal in mind, you are as adrift as a ship without a rudder. Here is an example:

Ellen has not gotten along with her roommate, Chris, for several weeks. Their relationship reached the crisis stage when, all in one evening, Chris left Ellen's hair

dryer on so it burned out, she spilled ink on the drawing
that Ellen had carefully prepared for her drafting class,
and she had a two-hour-and-forty-five-minute phone
conversation with her boyfriend, even though she knew
Ellen was expecting an important call. Ellen felt a mix-
ture of anxiety and rage. Her anxiety grew from her
realization that she could not afford an apartment on
her own and had not yet met any suitable roommates
because she had only been living in the city for three
months. Since Chris already knew her way around
town, Ellen had been counting on her for assistance in
getting to know the social and professional scenes, a
possibility that would be lost were their friendship to
end abruptly. On the other hand, she was angry because
she felt that Chris was exploiting the situation by intentionally making her feel that she only lived with Ellen
out of pity and therefore could walk all over her. Before
Ellen could decide how to respond, she had to choose a
goal: Should she end the relationship immediately or try
to preserve it? If she was interested in preserving it, she
must next decide how firm she should be in asking for
more consideration.

Ellen answered the first question by realizing that she
really did like Chris when the two of them were not stepping on each other's toes, and she realized that she had
much to gain from the relationship. She might also have
decided that the relationship was too much of a problem
to be worth the effort. She made her choice by using the
"one-by-four" table illustrated below. She examined
her thoughts about the rewards and costs of staying or
leaving, and placed a value on each entry, on a scale of 1
through 5, using 5 to indicate great importance and 1 to
indicate little importance. As you can see, she found 12
net value points for staying (21 reward points less 9 cost
points), and a negative 5 net value points for moving (9
potential reward points balanced against 14 potential
cost points). Given her perception of the various possible outcomes, she decided that it would be wisest for
her to stay and try to work things out. When you face
similar choices, you too might find it helpful to work

out your decision through use of this type of table, because it helps to make certain that you consider most if not all of the relevant factors, giving each its proper weight as you size things up at the moment.

Ellen's One-by-Four Decision-Making Table

If I stay				If I move			
Rewards	(Wt.)	Costs	(Wt.)	Rewards	(Wt.)	Costs	(Wt.)
Save money	5	Feel put down sometimes	4	Might find "perfect" roommate	5	Might end up with much worse roommate	5
Save hassle	3						
Get Chris's help	4	Lose some privacy due to Chris's borrowing	3	Could live closer to work	1	Would have to start over with new person; no energy for that now	5
Have a friend	5			Might find cheaper apartment	3		
Could learn to control my feelings better	4	Might feel I was giving in	2			Would have to buy some new furniture; Chris owns most things in apartment	4

Ellen next recognized that her feelings would be beyond control unless some change was achieved in the pattern of their interaction. To identify those changes, she made a list of things that she would like Chris to do, *not* a list of things that she wanted Chris to *stop* doing. For example, she wanted Chris to buy and use her own hair dryer, to work only at her own desk and drafting table, and to limit her use of the phone to 15 minutes per hour (as Ellen had been doing), so that calls could come in during 30 of every 60 minutes. In other words, she wanted Chris to respect her personal space much as she had been respecting Chris's right to privacy.

Once she knew her goals, Ellen was then ready to plan her approach. She decided to ask Chris to join her in an assessment of the first three months of their lives together, in order to identify changes that each could make to improve their interaction. She also decided that she should start the ball rolling by confessing that she knew she had regularly borrowed money from Chris and had been slow in repaying, and that she did play her radio too loudly when Chris was trying to sleep. It was her hope that her offering to make adjustments might elicit a comparable response from Chris.

Now she was ready to follow through. She chose a time that they normally enjoyed together—Saturday lunch while waiting for their clothes to be washed at the Laundromat—and put her plan to the test. The conversation lasted over an hour and concluded with a "want list" on which each wrote the changes she would like the other to make. They agreed *not* to promise to grant *all* of the requests at every opportunity, but to keep the list in mind and to do at least *some* of the things every day. While they walked back home, Ellen thoughtfully reviewed the events of the day and felt very pleased with herself because she had turned a troubled relationship into a secure one. Had the assessment come to a different conclusion, her task would have been to plan and execute a different approach to the achievement of the same worthwhile goals. She has taken important steps toward controlling her moods.

The process that Ellen followed illustrates one essential component of the planning process: problem solving with an action orientation. It involves five steps:

1. Selection of positive, specific goals
2. Formulation of a plan of action
3. Action on the plan
4. Assessment of the results
5. Formulation of alternative plans if the goals have not yet been achieved

We all go through these steps in attempting to find solutions to problems, even though we may not consciously use the number system. However, articulation of the steps each time we experience a troubling mood could lend great precision to our efforts to master many of the challenges we face.

Now we can turn to some specific techniques for promoting situation change and for developing greater skill in coping with negative moods.

Technique 1: A Break For R & R

Many of us lead unnecessarily pressured lives. We design schedules that are so tight that we have no pre-planned time to relax. As a result, we suffer from the ill effects of mounting tension and are much more likely to overact to the least frustration.

Playtime is not a luxury: it is a necessity for successful performance. Industry has increasingly recognized this fact by providing recreational opportunities at the sites of large factories and businesses. Large sums of money are being spent in the development of recreational opportunities that help workers to experience a change in pace through a break in routine. Relaxation of this sort discharges tension that interferes with creativity and productivity.

To keep within manageable bounds:

THINK THROUGH THE NORMAL ROUTINE
OF YOUR DAY TO FIND AN OPPORTUNITY
FOR AT LEAST ONE 30-MINUTE CHANGE OF PACE.

If your job involves sitting at a desk for eight hours, you might find a short walk invaluable. If you normally do physical jobs ranging from cleaning house to factory work, taking a sitting break to read a chapter from an interesting book, work on a crossword puzzle, chat with friends, or spend a little time on a hobby like macramé,

FIGURE 11.1

Planning and Monitoring Daily Rest Breaks

Day of Week	What are the times of your greatest normal strain?	When will you plan rest breaks to minimize your tension?	How will you use this time?
Monday			
Tuesday			
Wednesday			
Thursday			
Friday			
Saturday			
Sunday			

knitting, whittling, or sketching can all help to recoup your energy and calm your nerves.

Planning your breaks ahead of time is much better than waiting until exhaustion forces you to take a rest. When you plan ahead, your energy is likely to be consistently high because you know that a break is coming. When you push yourself to the breaking point your spirits are likely to be low and your performance poor. When you finally do slow down, you are not likely to feel that you have done the job well, which builds your tension even more.

In addition to deciding in advance just when you will take your breaks, it is a good idea to plan what you will do for relaxation. Be realistic in choosing the time and the activity. If you have the job of pushing husband and children out the door with breakfasts under their belts and lunch boxes under their arms, planning a break before the school bus arrives is unrealistic. In the same vein, if jogging is your pleasure, don't plan to spent the time writing an essay.

To help you with your planning, use the chart in Figure 11.1.

Technique 2: Meditation

Another way to cope with troublesome moods is meditation. This technique can help you to lower your general tension level and to exert control over many bodily processes. Armed with this control you can learn to relax as an alternative when you experience the urge to eat.

Meditation was first described in the Hindu *Vedas,* written between 1,000 and 500 years before the birth of Christ. Since that time, virtually every major religion has included meditation in its recommendations to the faithful.[5] As a modern technique in mood control, meditation has burst onto the contemporary scene as a haven for serenity seekers because its techniques are easily learned, readily followed, and very likely to produce good results.[6]

Meditation can be defined as the focusing of attention upon a single target such as an idea, a sound, or an aspect of physical functioning. When meditators achieve complete concentration upon one feature of their immediate experience, they are cleansed of their concerns with all other features. A cliché that well describes the effect of meditation is: *out of mind, out of body.*

Meditation is believed to produce a fourth level of consciousness. Waking, sleeping, and dreaming are the three levels of consciousness that are part of our normal life experience. The meditator is awake but all of his or her bodily processes appear to slow down temporarily: heart rate slows, oxygen consumption decreases, blood pressure lowers or at least stabilizes, electro-conductance of the skin decreases, and even brain waves change, with a decrease in beta waves and an increase in alpha waves. All of these meditation-produced changes are the opposite of reactions that are observed in connection with the urges to fight or flee.[5]

Successful meditation is a kind of mental cleansing. It involves achieving freedom from ordinary daily concerns by focusing one's attention upon a single idea. There are many ways of achieving this result. In transcendental meditation one relaxes and simply repeats over and over the personal "mantra" that has been learned from a trainer. Less ritualized meditation instruction involves simply repeating a word such as "one" over and over. Zen meditation involves a noncritical reflection on the emotions and events that one has experienced during the preceding hours or day. This reflection must be "detached and nonevaluative," as it is intended not as a form of self-analysis but as a technique for achieving an important level of self-acceptance. This kind of nonevaluative self-reflection is difficult to achieve because one constantly evaluates the extent to which he or she is nonevaluative, a paradox that must be overcome if the fourth level of consciousness is to be achieved. Finally, meditators sometimes focus their attention on an external stimulus—they may focus their eyes on a candle or a flower, or close their eyes while listening to a quiet, repetitive sound such as a low hum or tick.

Would-be meditators would do well to try all of these techniques—a single-syllable word frequently repeated, nonevaluative review of recent experience, focusing on a visual object or a repetitious sound—in order to find the most comfortable means of purging their consciousness of troublesome concerns. There is no right or wrong in choosing one or more of these approaches; the only acceptable criterion is one's own feelings of emotional comfort and control.

Meditation is practiced for periods of approximately fifteen to twenty minutes in the most quiet and calm environment available. Choose a time each day and make an effort to practice every day. The meditator sits in a comfortable position with head and arms supported. The meditator breathes through the nose and begins by concentrating on the process of breathing by mentally repeating a word such as "one" with every exhale. When intrusive thoughts occur, the meditator simply retreats from them. There is no active fight against preoccupations: instead, there is simply a greater concentration upon the word, the effort to recount the day's experience, the point in space, or the sound in the air.

It is neither difficult nor easy to meditate. The achievement of the fourth level of meditative consciousness requires practice, and successful practice in turn requires routine. Therefore, it is important for each person to choose a time of day when meditation will be practiced and to make it a point to practice meditating at this same time every day.

Technique 3: Training Yourself So That Your Negative Thoughts Don't Get the Best of You

It has long been known that our emotional reactions have two components: an idea that is coupled with a physical reaction. Sometimes we can have an idea that passes without notice, but at other times that same idea can trigger a strong emotional response. If we can train ourselves to respond to troubling ideas without physical tension, we can protect ourselves from the ravages of uncontrolled emotion. As Dr. Joseph Wolpe of Temple University was to discover, this self-training is possible if we learn to relax our bodies at will and then to visualize thoughts while we are relaxed.[6]

Successful physical relaxation depends upon getting to know the way in which your body experiences tension. Sit in a quiet place or lie on a smooth surface.

Begin by taking a few deep breaths and exhaling slowly. Think about the air passing into your lungs as you inhale. Then become aware of the feeling of the air slowly escaping through your nose as you exhale. Three or four deep breaths will prepare you for the process of bringing your muscles under control.

Close your eyes and concentrate all of your energy on one muscle group after another. If you are right-handed, begin always with your left hand and foot. If you are left-handed, begin with the right hand and foot. Start by pointing one toe and stretching your leg fully from the hip, tightening your thigh and calf muscles. You should feel a slight wedge sensation in the arch of your foot and a pulling of the muscles in your stomach and back as your leg stretches. Sense the complete feeling and then relax the tension. Focus all of your attention on the feeling of relaxation. Then repeat the exercise with the other foot.

Next make a fist with your nondominant hand while stretching your arm and contracting the muscles in your forearm and biceps. Hold this position for a few seconds as you concentrate upon the sensation of tension, then try to have your consciousness enter the muscles of your shoulder, arm, and hand as they relax. Repeat this exercise with the other hand.

Then focus your attention upon your stomach and buttocks. Tighten all of the muscles in your lower body, hold them for a few seconds as you concentrate upon the sensation. Then relax the muscles slowly while you continue to study the feelings of relaxation.

Repeat the same sequence with your upper body muscles, "hunching" your shoulders as you contract your chest muscles. Notice the involvement of your upper arms and stomach as you feel the upper body tense. Then concentrate on the feeling of these muscles as they relax.

Finally, concentrate on the muscles of your lips, cheeks, and forehead. Screw up your face tightly and try to feel every wrinkle as you hold your tense expression for a few seconds. Then slowly release the tension.

When you have gone through a period of tensing each muscle group for about five seconds and then spent about fifteen seconds gradually relaxing the muscles and concentrating on the absence of tension, your limbs should feel heavier and you should experience a kind of sagging of your body onto the floor. If you still feel tension in any muscle group, repeat the exercise for that group and then each of the succeeding groups beginning with legs, then arms, lower body, upper body, and head, in that order.

When you feel fully relaxed, try to focus your attention on a specific area of your body at random: penetrate that area with your consciousness and fully experience the sensation of relaxation of that area. The goal of this relaxation exercise is to train you to be able to identify both tension and relaxation so that you can learn to instruct yourself to relax, wherever you are, when you begin to feel tension arising.

Once you have learned to relax, you are ready to begin to train yourself to induce this same calm feeling at times when you might otherwise respond with strong emotions. While you are relaxed, try to imagine yourself interacting with people who normally "make you feel tense." See yourself calmly responding first to meeting these people and then to interactions that involve increasing challenge. Any time that you experience the telltale sign of physical tension, back off, relax yourself again, and make a new attempt. *Never allow yourself to become tense while you are practicing relaxation training.* Eventually, you will have an imprint in your mind of you responding to would-be troubling situations with self-assurance and calm.

When you find yourself in these situations, summon up the image of the tranquil you and silently instruct yourself to relax those parts of your body that are your normal tension centers. You may still experience some emotion: that is only normal. You should, however, find that your emotions are now within your control and that you are free to handle the situation with assertive action.

IN A NUTSHELL

Anxiety, depression, boredom, anger, and stress are four emotions that very often trigger a vicious cycle of tension/eating/more tension/more eating. You can passively accept these emotions or you can actively attempt to deal with them. You can begin mood control by choosing facilitative labels for the events that concern you. You can go on by carefully structuring major decisions in a problem-solving framework. Then you can interrupt the cycle at an early point by assertively trying to change your interaction with others. You can also have a second line of defense by training yourself to plan rest periods that will keep your energy high, by learning to meditate to achieve a generalized tension control, and by learning to relax away interfering emotions when specific situations arise. All of these techniques can help to build your mastery over your moods and thereby cut back one source of the pressure that builds your urge to eat.

CHAPTER 12

Sleep Control: Another Mood-Management Technique

SLEEP. YOU SPENT about one-third of your life doing it. You devote about one-third of your living space to it. You take it for granted until it goes awry and then it can destroy your functioning for days on end. Because it affects the way you feel, it can have a profound effect upon the way that you eat. But you have probably never thought of using sleep control as a means of gaining mastery over your urge to eat.

For the ancient Greeks, Sleep and Death were brother gods who dwelt in the regions of Hell. When a Greek passed into the realm of sleep, he entrusted himself to the gods, who might claim his soul for all eternity. Therefore, to sleep was to venture behind the mists of an awesome unknown.[1]

Some mystery still surrounds the nature and functions of sleep despite our use of fancy electronics to probe its every dimension. Many bodily functions slow down during sleep including muscular activity, heart rate, body temperature, and metabolic rate. We even consume about a fifth less oxygen when sleeping as opposed to being awake. While common sense tells us that sleep is a time to "recharge our batteries," the slowing down of all our functions would hardly permit this worthy chore to be accomplished.[2]

Laboratory researchers have shown that there are five different stages of sleep. Brain waves differ at each of these stages. The first stage is closest to our waking brain-wave pattern, the fourth is the slowest and least like our waking pattern. We go from stage 1 to 2 to 3 to 4, then back to 2 again when we are undisturbed. From stage 2 we go into the fifth or Rapid Eye Movement (REM) stage, and it is during this stage that our dreams take place. Half of our sleep time is spent in stage 2 and about one-fifth is spent in the dream or REM stage. The rest of our sleep time is divided more or less equally between stages 1, 3, and 4. If our sleep is interrupted during the REM, third, or fourth stage, we seem to make up the difference during the nights that follow. Therefore it is not necessary for us to have the same amount of total sleep time every night: what we strive for is the proper amount of REM and deep sleep.[3]

Disturbances in sleep cycles appear to be more uncomfortable than changes in the absolute amount of sleep. Most people, if placed in a room in which cues that indicate the time of day are removed, adjust to a pattern that is very similar to their normal sleep cycle. When subjects are asked to go to sleep three hours before or after their normal bedtime, they show considerable behavioral and psychological disorganization. Performance of tasks which require concentration deteriorates markedly and mood generally turns toward irritability and depression. These are common experiences of air-travelers on transmeridian trips. Those flying three or more hours to the east have greater adjustment difficulties than those flying similar distances west because the deterioration associated with falling asleep earlier than usual is greater than that associated with falling asleep later.

Most travelers find that they require anywhere from one to seven days to readjust their sleep rhythms. Thus, even after a night or two of normal sleep following a night of sleep disruption, judgment may be poorer than normal. Therefore, it is a good idea to postpone the need to make important decisions for at least forty-eight hours following any long-distance flight.[4]

People with sleep disturbances often complain of difficulty in falling asleep at night. On the average they have been found to spend close to an hour awake in bed before falling asleep for the first time. They also report waking up an average of two or three times per night, and they are more likely than good sleepers to complain about restlessness through the night and waking up with the birds. Despite the fact that they spend fewer hours asleep at night, they sleep on the average only about an hour less than good sleepers, making up for some of their lost sleep by catnaps during the day. Also, as suggested earlier, they have about as much stage 3 and 4 and REM-stage sleep as good sleepers, giving up some time from the more shallow second stage of sleep.[5]

The major problem faced by insomniacs—those who sleep less than six and a half hours per night, who spend at least thirty minutes falling asleep, who are awake for at least half an hour during the night, and who experience great fatigue during the day—is not so much their lack of sleep as the fact that their sleep seems to be chronically *deregulated*. In other words, it is the unpredictability of when they will fall asleep and when they will wake up rather than the amount of sleep time lost during their twisting and turning episodes that contributes to their daytime problems.

Not surprisingly, their daytime problems are many. Insomniacs perform certain attention-demanding tasks more poorly than good sleepers. They also complain about emotional problems ranging from chronic tension and mild depression to exaggerated concern about bodily functions. Increased heart symptoms, elevated blood pressure, and regular and severe tension headaches are other common complaints among poor sleepers.[6] Unfortunately, many people turn to food as a means of coping with each of these stresses.

While a definite relationship between body weight and sleep irregularity has *not* been found,[7] there is good evidence that loss of sleep and overeating do go hand in hand. When sleep is irregular, mood changes for the worse. When mood is bad, many people turn to food for solace, as has been said. But when bad moods are coupled with fatigue that has been brought on by sleep loss, the resort to food is more likely still.[8]

It has been shown, for example, that many people turn to food as a replacement for sleep. It has also been shown that when sleep is very disturbed, individuals suffering from anorexia nervosa (a serious psychological problem in which people have been known to starve themselves to death) tend to eat less while overweight people tend to eat more. Conversely, a return to normal sleep is likely to be coupled with weight gain by anorexics and weight loss by the obese.[9] Therefore, the regulation of disturbed sleep is an important step to be taken in any weight-management program.

Sizing Up Your Sleep Patterns

Many people overestimate the amount of difficulty which they have in sleeping while underestimating the amount of sleep which they get. Therefore, the best way to obtain a good measure of your sleeping pattern is to complete the data in Figure 12:1 for the next seven days. Getting into and out of bed at more or less the same time, whether for nighttime or nap sleep, helps to regulate your sleep. Therefore, assessment of these behaviors is important in adding up your sleeping quotient. Other important elements include limiting your fluid, coffee, and alcohol consumption, learning not to use the bed as a place for all manner of activities that could and should be done elsewhere, and making an attempt to be physically and psychologically relaxed before retiring. These are the kinds of behaviors that you will monitor in using Figure 12.1.

After seven days of recordkeeping you can add up your sleep score as follows:

For Question 1: Did you go to bed within the same one-hour range (e.g., between 10:30 and 11:30) at least six of the seven nights? If so, give yourself 10 points. If not, score nothing.

For Question 2: Did you fall asleep within fifteen minutes of going to bed at least six of the seven nights? If so, give yourself 5 points: if not, deduct 1 point for each night in which you tossed and turned for longer than fifteen minutes.

For Question 3: Did you manage not to look at the clock before daylight at least six of the seven nights? If so, give yourself 5 points: if not, deduct 1 point for each night that you checked the time before dawn.

For Question 4: Did you plan to wake up after the same number of hours of sleep at least six of the seven nights? If so, give yourself 5 points. If not, score nothing.

For Question 5: Did you wake up within thirty minutes of the same time on at least six of the seven days (e.g., between 7:00 and 7:30). If so, give yourself 5 points; if not, deduct 1 point for each morning more than one that you woke up at a time outside of your normal range.

For Question 6: Did you get out of bed within thirty minutes of waking up at least six mornings out of seven? If so, you have earned another 5 points. If not, deduct 1 point for each morning that you lingered in bed for longer than half an hour.

For Questions 7, 8, 9, 11: Score 1 point for each time that you could answer each of these questions "yes."

For Question 10: Score 5 points if you took no naps or if you took a nap for approximately the same amount of time at about the same hour every day. Deduct 1 point for each time that you took an unusually long or an unscheduled nap because you were overtired.

Sixty is a top score in this inventory, and it will be earned by good sleepers who do two things:

FIGURE 12.1

A Sleep Evaluation Record

	Monday	Tuesday	Wednes-day	Thursday	Friday	Saturday	Sunday	Total Points
1. What time did you get into bed?								
2. Approximately what time did you fall asleep?								
3. How many times did you wake up long enough to check the time during the night?								
4. What time did you plan to wake up?								
5. What time did you actually wake up?								
6. What time did you get out of bed?								
7. In the morning after breakfast, did you feel well rested?								

8. Did you feel well rested midday?						
9. Did you feel well rested in the late afternoon?						
10. How many minutes did you spend napping during the day?						
11. Did you feel particularly tired before getting into bed for the night?						
TOTAL POINTS						

1. They determine how many hours of sleep they need per night; and
2. They get this sleep at highly regular hours.

Our need for sleep appears to be highly individual. A study in England showed that one in twelve people studied slept under five hours nightly, while 15 percent reported sleeping five to six hours, 62 percent for seven to eight hours, and 15 percent for nine or more hours per night.[10]

Americans sleep an average of 7.5 hours per night, we wake up once during the night about four nights out of ten, and we are efficient sleepers, snoring away for about 88 percent of our time in bed. However, the older we are, the less efficiently we sleep and women report more sleep restlessness than men.[11] Cases have been reported in which a single hour of sleep was sufficient for years on end,[12] while others may require nightly sleep of ten hours or more.

On you can determine your own sleep needs and you can do this by keeping track of your sleep time at night and your energy and mood by day, eventually finding the proper balance. Once you know the amount of sleep you need to keep going, you must regulate the hours of sleep. Remembering that daily circadian rhythms influence everything that we experience during the day, you can appreciate the fact that sleeping regular hours can help you to achieve a well-regulated rhythm to your life. Therefore, 15 points or 25 percent of your total sleep inventory score can be earned through sleep regularity.

Another third of the points that you can earn in measuring the adequacy of your sleep results from your feelings of alertness or fatigue throughout the day (question 7, 8, 9, and 11). You may be "tired" at various times of the day because your work or play does not interest you or because your diet is inadequate. But if you find that you are tired at different times of the day throughout the seven days of the week, the chances are that you are experiencing the effects of inadequate sleep. Therefore, a score of 15 or less on these questions indicates a need for better sleep management.

Finally, difficulty in falling asleep (question 2) or in getting out of bed (question 6), and taking of irregular naps (question 10), are all further indications of a sleep problem. Less than optimal scores on these three questions pose further evidence that you are undermining your own functioning by mismanaging your sleep.

Steps in Sleep Management

If you have a chronic sleep problem, it is a good idea to have a complete medical checkup. There are at least thirty-two different causes of sleep problems ranging from simply corrected difficulties such as a poor sleep environment to illnesses and serious diseases. It is important to make certain that your sleep difficulties are not caused by an untreated illness. Because of its interdependence with basic biological processes, disturbances in sleep can be a symptom of some underlying illness and this possibility should be eliminated before you take steps to improve the quality of your sleep.[13]

A Five-Step Program of Sleep Control

When you have a clean bill of health, make a decision about how you will approach your sleep problem. One approach would be to take a sleeping drug, generally termed a "hypnotic" drug. Use of these "sleeping pills" is very widespread. Americans spend $100 million for prescription drugs alone each year, with hundreds of millions more for over-the-counter drugs. Unfortunately, use of these drugs has been found to *increase rather than decrease* sleep problems. You feel tired so you take a pill. Over time, you develop a "tolerance" to the drug—your usual dose loses its effect—so you increase the dose you take. Higher doses of the drug cause disruption of your sleep rhythms so you feel chronically fatigued. That leads you to take higher doses still, to develop a dependence upon the drug, and to join the legions who have made sleeping pills one of America's most seriously abused drugs.[14]

Once the decision has been made to develop sleep control without the use of drugs, the next step is to reduce emotional and physical tension before you retire for the night. Managing your moods (Chapter 11) and increasing your physical activity (Chapter 14) can help you in this regard.[15]

Now you are ready to begin your sleep-control regime. Now many hours of sleep do you need, as determined by your use of the sleep inventory? Because many people *overestimate* the amount of time that they spend trying to fall asleep and then *underestimate* the amount of time that they actually spend sleeping, adjustments in sleep time of thirty to sixty minutes are often sufficient.

Knowing how much sleep you should have, next decide that you will:

1. Go to bed at exactly *the same time of night,* seven nights each week.
2. Set the alarm to *wake up at exactly the same time every morning of the week,* no matter how long you tossed and turned before falling asleep the night before; and
3. Do not take naps if you can avoid them, but if you must nap, do so at *exactly the same time every day.*

This program offers the same gains and presents the same challenges as regulating the time of your urges to eat (Chapter 9). In both instances you will be attempting to retrain your body to move from chaotic to controlled biorhythmic functioning. As with your eating regulations, once you have gotten your sleep under control, you will be able to tolerate a little flexibility in your hours of retiring and waking. To achieve control of a process that has been deregulated for months or years requires close attention consistency. Therefore, in your initial efforts at sleep control, perfection should be your goal, as it is with retiming your urges to eat.

The second step of the program is another measure that you must take to help you sleep through the night. Very often people wake up at night because their bladders are full or because their bodies are reacting to signals from stimulants or depressants. Therefore:

1. Try to drink as little as possible at 4 P.M.;
2. Limit your consumption of coffee and tea as much as possible during the day, and have neither after 4 P.M.; and
3. Do not drink any alcoholic beverage, day or night.

As you will recall, these were some of the behaviors that you monitored in determining your sleep quotient. Curbing your fluid intake after 4 P.M. will help to make certain that your bladder is empty after you retire. Cutting down on coffee, tea, and alcohol will help you to relax more at bedtime. It is, of course, well recognized that coffee and tea are stimulants (tea has about half as much caffeine as coffee). But many people consider alcohol a "pick-me-up" by day and a drink to "calm me down" by night. In fact, the exact functions of alcohol are not fully understood but it is generally regarded as a central nervous system depressant. When alcohol enters the body, the nervous system steps up its activity to make up for alcohol's inhibiting effects. When the alcohol is burned off, the central nervous system is still overactive. This explains the tremors experienced by chronic drinkers when their intake slacks off. But even social drinkers experience this delayed arousal effect which can lead to sleep disturbance and tension that makes falling asleep again quite difficult.

The third step concerns management of the stimulus conditions of sleep.[16] In Chapter 7 it was pointed out that overeaters often condition themselves to feel hunger when they have linked eating and certain kinds of non-food-related activities such as watching television. In these instances, the television set, the reading matter, or the work project can become conditioned

cues for the urge to eat. When poor sleepers use their
beds for many different activities, it is possible that
rather than cueing sleep, the bed can become a conditioned stimulus for other kinds of reactions. While it
has been shown that good and poor sleepers both do
about the same number of nonsleep activities, like reading or watching TV—even eating in bed—those with
sleeping problems may be less able to tolerate this poor
conditioning. Therefore it is important to:

> TRY TO MAKE SLEEP ROUTINES
> A "PURE EXPERIENCE"
> JUST AS YOU DID WITH EATING.

For example, the television set should be turned
around so that it cannot be watched from bed (or, better
still, removed from the bedroom) and reading should be
done in a chair rather than in bed. Activities such as sex
which normally (but not necessarily) take place in bed
should be given their own unique cues. For example,
using a special light reserved only for sex, or lying with
heads at the foot of the bed instead of in the normal
sleeping position can both help to dissociate other activities from bed and allow the bed to become a pure
stimulus for rest.

In addition to retraining yourself to associate only
rest with bed, it is also important to eliminate *or lessen
other distractors in the bedroom*. For example, controlling the level of light with room darkeners can be
helpful. Use of an inexpensive "white noise" machine
can help to mask distracting sounds. These are small
devices which are sold by drug and department stores
and they can be highly effective in muting the impact of
sleep-disturbing sounds.

Another help is a program of muscle relaxation.[17] As
you will recall, this program (described on pages
140–142) calls for tensing and relaxing major muscle
groups beginning with the legs, then the arms, lower
body, upper body, and head and neck. Because you cannot be tense and relaxed at the same time, training in

relaxation can bring your bodily stress under control, and the method has been very effective in helping insomniacs to become more sleep-efficient.

Step five calls for thought control. The myriad thoughts that cross your mind as you try to fall asleep provoke emotional tension that bar the door to relaxing sleep. Therefore, efforts to break up the obsessional grip of such thoughts can go far toward overcoming this sleep-delaying tension.

Thought purging can be accomplished by concentrating on neutral ideas. The familiar counting of sheep is not far from the mark. Recitation of a formula or concentration upon pleasing colors, sensations, and experiences can also do the trick, as can listening to soft music. However you focus your ideas, it is important to find a stimulus that is sufficiently strong to take your mind away from anxiety about whether or not you are falling asleep, and away from the major preoccupations of your life.

Follow the five-step program for a week. You may find it necessary to adapt one or more of the recommendations to your personal lifestyle. In adjusting the program to your individual needs, be certain to keep in mind the importance of consistency in all of your sleep rituals. This point cannot be overstated! The chart in Figure 12.2 is intended to help you keep track of your sleep-control efforts. Fill it out daily as a means of giving yourself feedback about what you have done and the jobs which still must be attended to. After a week, reassess your sleep adequacy by answering the questions in Figure 12.1 again. If you score higher on this second administration of the chart, you know that you are heading in the right direction. If you show no change, you should renew your efforts to find the proper combination of mood management, exercise (see Chapter 14), scheduling, stimulus control, and physical- and thought-control mechanisms so that you can enjoy the restorative sleep which we all need to function at our best.

FIGURE 12.2

Record of Success in the Sleep-Management Program

	Monday	Tuesday	Wednes- day	Thurs- day	Friday	Saturday	Sunday
1. Did you get into bed on schedule?							
2. Did you get out of bed on schedule?							
3. Did you schedule your naps and sleep only when planned?							
4. Did you reduce your fluid intake after 4 P.M.?							
5. Did you refrain from coffee or tea after 4 P.M.?							

6. Did you reduce your alcohol consumption?						
7. Did you remember to use the bed only for sleep (unless you associated another activity such as sex with a special set of cues)?						
8. Did you physically relax yourself upon getting into bed?						
9. Did you concentrate on neutral thoughts, avoiding preoccupation with falling asleep or with the cares of your waking life?						

IN A NUTSHELL

Many different factors affect our moods and our eating behavior. One of these factors is the level of our energy or, its opposite, our fatigue. If we suffer from irregular sleep, our moods are likely to be sour and our energy low. Sleep disturbance is very common in America and it is a self-made disorder. We can gain control of our sleep by retraining ourselves in regular sleep patterns and in actively managing our sleeping environment. Improve your sleep and you can improve your mood. Improve your mood and you can curb another source of your urge to eat more than you should.

CHAPTER 13

Hindrances and Help
from Members of
Your Family

IF YOU SEE an overweight man on the street, what are
the chances that he will be married to a heavy woman?
Excellent, according to data collected in the Ten State
Nutrition Survey. Dr. Stanley Garn of the University of
Michigan has analyzed these data carefully and has
found that whether or not heavy men and women marry
one another, over the course of their lives together the
leaner of the two will gradually put on extra weight to
match the proportions of the heavier spouse. When
Mother Goose observed that "Jack Spratt can eat no
fat,/ His wife can eat no lean,/ And so between the two
of them,/ They licked the platter clean," she naturally
had in mind couples in the early days of their lives
together. Because over the years, they will both lean
toward the fat.[1]

Can the same be said of the fat child? What are the
chances that a heavy child will have a heavy sibling? Dr.
Garn found that if one child of two is heavy, there is a
40 percent chance that the other will be heavy as well. If
the fat child is one of three, there is an 80 percent chance

that one of the other two will also be fat. As you might
expect by now, there is also about a 75 percent chance
that the fat child, whom you single out on the street,
will have at least one overweight parent.[2]

For many years it was believed that these findings of
fatness similarities among family members meant that
overweight was under the control of genetics. But an im-
pressive array of findings has weakened this belief. It
has been learned, for example, that genetically caused
obesities are rare, and that when they occur they are
usually accompanied by a variety of other anomalies
such as skeletal malformations and mental retardation.
Moreover, it has been learned that genes generally influence *body frame size* but they do not often directly
influence *fat patterning per se*.[3]

While genetics play a factor in determining the predisposition to be heavy or lean, our genes receive important assistance in their mission from our experience
after birth. This finding is supported by two groups of
studies. In one it was shown that twins who are reared
together are very similar in height and weight while
twins who are separated at birth are similar in height but
not in weight. In the second group of studies it was
shown that foster and adopted children bear the same
degree of resemblance to their new parents as do other
children toward their natural parents.[4] Shared eating
and exercise activities within the family thus seem to
give the genes a major assist in making family members
look-alikes.

Mothers are often signaled out as the arch-villains
because they are believed to be the architects of their
children's obesity. But the Ten State Nutrition Survey
data indicated fathers as well. Parents and children in
the ten states were shown to have the following parent-
child correlations in body weight:

Father-son	.25
Father-daughter	.20
Mother-son	.26
Mother-daughter	.19

Therefore, fathers and mothers seem to have about the same impact upon the eating and activity patterns of their children, although both have greater influence upon their sons than upon their daughters.

Mothers do have primary control over their newborn's feeding patterns. While some babies come into life with an above average number of cells in which fat can be stored, many babies who are overfed during the early weeks and months of their lives develop an unusually high number of these cells. As the child matures, these cells fill up with fat and increase in size. It is believed by many that the cells create a chemical need for fat and that if they are fat deprived, the body is "out-of-balance" and strives to correct the balance by excess food intake.[5] The evidence on this point is not at all clear, however, and it is probably safest to conclude that overfeeding infants can lead to a predisposition to fatness in childhood, adolescence, and later life, but that this predisposition requires a helping hand from weight-related learning later on along the line.

It has been estimated that about 70 percent of the infants under one year range from being overweight to being obese. And yet only about 49 percent of the ten-year-olds are overweight or obese. About one-third of those who were very heavy babies are still very heavy at the age of seven while 60 percent of the seven-year-olds who are very heavy were overweight at birth. Therefore, some children whom one would expect to be genetically doomed to obesity at birth have a different experience in life. Interestingly, these tend to be children in larger families. As one researcher put it, "A mother with only one child is more concerned with persuading that one child to eat and grow than is a mother with several children."[6] Of course, it is also possible that with more than one mouth to feed there may simply not be enough food to go round to fatten all of the family's young.

When the dust settles, it becomes clear that, as the animal husbandry experts have learned, it is possible to breed animals for fatness. But the fattening process can be helped along by overfeeding the cultured animals and by keeping them as inactive as possible. There is no reason to believe that humans are any different. Some people have an inherited predisposition to fatness. But the effects of this predisposition can be mitigated to some extent by careful dietary management and by concerted attempts to increase the rate of energy expenditure.

The Forces That Fatten Children

Unfortunately, the false idea that "one cannot overfeed an infant" dies as slowly as the utterly foolish belief that "a fat baby is a healthy baby."[7]

In infancy the mother clearly has control of what the baby eats. During childhood, the youngster can become a co-conspirator with his or her mother but still the mother calls most of the nutritional shots. By adolescence, however, the teenager has an opportunity to make many independent eating decisions. Some of these decisions may not be wise. It is a fact that overweight teenagers are far more likely than their normal-weight classmates to have highly erratic eating patterns. Overweight adolescents are the ones most likely to report skipping breakfast and lunch and to have ill-defined mealtimes in general. Their food intake is also most likely to vary significantly in content and quantity from one day to the next.[8]

Overweight children are also more likely than their normal-weight peers to come from families in which there is some interpersonal disturbance that may or may not involve the use of food directly. For example, mothers of the overweight have been shown to have been more likely to use food as rewards for good behavior and the families of the overweight were much less likely to use mealtimes as times of family closeness. In addition, family and marital strife which often led to temporary or permanent parental separations was also the more common lot of the overweight. Finally, whether the family stresses were overt or covert, the nutritional practices of the teenagers tended to be quite poor if family tension was high and good if family interaction was positive.[9]

Unfortunately, it is not known whether family stress came before or after the development of adolescents' weight problem. Moreover, it is very important to point out that some, but by no means all of the families of overweight adolescents displayed these stressful reactions. In fact, some of the families of heavy teenagers can be considered to be among the better or even best functioning of families.

A third difference found between overweight and normal-weight teenagers is the *amount and intensity of their physical activity*. In every study to date, normal-weight adolescents were found to exercise longer and more vigorously than their heavier classmates. While it has been observed that most Americans spend far more time eating than exercising, overweight adolescents seem to use what little time they spend exercising quite inefficiently. For example, slow-motion movies of girls at a summer camp found slim campers were 150 percent more active than overweight campers while playing volleyball and 250 percent more active while swimming.[10] These frequently reported results stand in sharp contrast to the studies of teenage eating habits showing that overweight teenagers consume about the same amount of food as their slender classmates. One significant key to the control of teenage obesity, therefore, is a carefully planned increase in the level of physical activity, step by step.

It is by no means clear whether inactivity or overweight comes first. However, there is evidence that activity patterns are learned along with eating habits early in the young child's life and, of course, their parents and siblings are the unwitting teachers. Whether inactivity or overeating comes first, it is clear that by definition the overweight take in more energy than they burn, and they store their excess energy as fat.[11] The longer this problem persists for children and adolescents, the stronger will be the habits that can lock the child into a lifelong pattern of excess weight. Because 80 percent of the adolescents who are overweight face obesity in adulthood,[12] prudence demands that, whenever possible, the chain which leads to obesity must be broken at its very earliest possible point.

In many households this requires rethinking decisions about infant feeding practices, decisions about early-childhood activity patterns, decisions about the family's social use of food, and decisions about the food and exercise options offered to adolescents.[13]

Some Very Important Considerations

Decades of research have led to the following conclusions about the role of family experience in promoting and maintaining obesity:

1. For a small number of individuals, genetic and metabolic factors do create a predisposition to above average fatness.
2. For most people, however, the foundation for fatness is laid down after birth.
3. Infant overfeeding, childhood inactivity, erratic food habits in adolescence, family tension, and spousal influence all contribute to a situation in which the overweight simply consume more food energy than they burn, *even though their eating may not be excessive in the least*.

Therefore, *social learning* plays a major role in the development of obesity, a role which may be far more important than that of biological factors which have received so much attention in the past.

It is reasonable to assume that few people in this culture choose to be fat. This fatness must be viewed as a consequence of the interaction between biology and experience, neither of which were under the direct control of the overweight person during the most important early, formative years. This leads to the further assumption that

> *NO PERSON WHO HAS BEEN HEAVY SINCE BIRTH*
> *OR EARLY CHILDHOOD WAS THE ARCHITECT OF*
> *HIS OR HER OWN OBESITY. BUT IT IS ALSO ESSENTIAL*
> *TO REALIZE THAT, IN THE FINAL ANALYSIS,*
> *IT IS ONLY THE OVERWEIGHT PERSON WHO CAN*
> *DECIDE THAT CORRECTIVE ACTION IS NECESSARY.*
> *WHILE HE OR SIIE DID NOT CHOOSE FATNESS,*
> *IT IS THE OVERWEIGHT PERSON*
> *WHO MUST CHOOSE THINNESS.*

This leads to the inescapable conclusion that each person must make a personal decision to gain or lose weight. No matter how good their motivation might be, failure in weight loss is the only reasonable expectation when others attempt to make this most important decision. In fact, when parents or spouses attempt to impose this decision, relationships can become so strained that greater weight gain results.

Let's see how this might look in real life. Jenny is fifteen. When she was born she was a "bouncy baby." As an infant she was covered with soft and cuddly "baby fat." She was "plump" as a child, "husky" as a preteen, and "on the heavy side" in mid-adolescence. Through most of this time she has weighed about 25 percent more than she should. Her mother is "on the stout side" and her father is slowly moving from a size 36 to a size 38 belt. Both parents know that Jenny's weight is a problem. Her father becomes angry when he sees her overeat, her mother feels a sting of pain when she sees Jenny reach for extra cake or cookies. Both parents bring sweets into the house, "for company," "to celebrate this or that," or "just to keep Jenny happy." Both also eat the sweets that they bring home.

Jenny feels hopeless about her weight. She used to be made fun of by the other children on the block, but now she is accepted although not warmly welcomed into their activities. She tried to play the active games the other play but had a hard time keeping up, so she spent much of the game time alone. She does not like to see her body in the mirror, although she does like her pretty face and smooth complexion. She feels hassled by her parents about her weight and resists their attempts to make her thin. Basically, she resents their efforts to control her weight because she is struggling to find her own boundaries for her own sense of self and she feels their efforts to be encroachments on her personal life space. Although she has never said anything about it, she also doubts their sincerity: "If weight control is so important, why are they so fat? and why do they eat the junk they do?"

What, then, is the role of Jenny's parents? Whether or not they contributed to the development of her inactivity and overeating, they can play an important role in her development of more constructive patterns of behavior. Jenny will have to come to her own decision about whether or not to lose weight. Her parents can help her to identify the problem and the possible solutions, but she alone must make the commitment to change.

Once she has made the decision, her parents, her brothers and sisters, and even her friends, can all cooperate to make her weight change possible. This help begins from the realization that all family members have an important impact upon each other's behavior:

1. They set examples for each other;
2. They *prompt* each other's actions; and
3. They selectively *pay off* each other's efforts.

Everything that is said or done in a family serves as an example for others. If Jenny sees Dad take a third helping of spaghetti, she learns that three are not too many servings of Mom's pasta. When Dad sees Mom take a modest first portion and decline seconds, he learns that she values moderation. When Mom sees Jenny take an apple instead of a cupcake for dessert, that, too, is an object lesson. We always display our values to others by what we do rather than by what we say!

Family members also prompt each other's actions both by word and deed. Mom reminds Junior to drink his milk—that's a verbal prompt. She also keeps the freezer well supplied with Junior's favorite flavor of ice cream—that's a prompt by deed. When we are not busy demonstrating the kind of behavior which we expect, we are usually occupied with promoting its occurrence, directly or indirectly.

Finally, family members also follow one another's actions with some kind of response which may either strengthen or weaken chances that the same action will be repeated another time. The most powerful and also the most common kind of payoff is attention. Attention is a universally powerful way of strengthening behavior. People will imperil their lives to gain attention, and children would rather be punished than be ignored. Therefore, any response made to another's action will make that action more likely to be repeated.

Everything that members of the family do has an impact upon everything done by the others. Sometimes the impact is exactly what is expected; sometimes the predictions are proven dead wrong. Right or wrong, positive or negative, family members cannot *not* influence one another.[14]

Therefore, in order to be as helpful as possible:

1. Every member of the family must set the best *example* possible;
2. Each must take responsibility for *prompting* the actions which he or she considers important; and
3. Each must consistently *pay off the others* for their constructive actions.

How Parents Can Help a Teenager Lose Weight and Maintain the Loss

The typical adolescent doubles in weight during the teenage years. This growth is obviously a time of great importance for a healthy adulthood. Important, too, is the fact that much of the weight gain of teenagers is at-

…e to an excess of food intake over energy ex-
…e, and not simply the result of overeating.
…ogether, these observations require that:

1. Goals of very gradual weight loss be established for
   teenagers;
2. The nutritional needs of developing bodies be met completely; and
3. A well-balanced food plan be combined with a gradual
   increase in activity.

Rapid weight loss due to excessive cuts in the minimum food requirements and radically increased exercise
can create greater problems than they could possibly
solve. The name of the game for both children and
adults is *weight loss through small steps*.

Parents can start the ball rolling by developing some
very important attitudes. They must give up the idea
that fat children are healthy children. They must also
give up the belief that the average, healthy child suffers
injury through overheating and fatigue after vigorous
exercise. In addition, they must give up the time-hon-
ored cliché that "parents know best." Such thinking is
a red flag to the emerging adolescent.

Attempts of parents to hold the reins too tightly
generally lead to rebellion. For example, parents who
peer over their child's shoulder at the readout on the
bathroom scale every day are likely to find the numbers
growing ever worse. A sensible weight-management
program for teenagers must fully credit the child's in-
dependence and capacity to take responsibility.

Parents should openly discuss the caloric facts with
their children. For example, it is a fact that just two
extra cookies per day (e.g., chocolate chip or fig bars)
can add up to 700 extra calories per week and to over ten
unwanted pounds per year. It is also true that a half-
hour walk can burn about 150 calories per day, 4,500
per month, or 54,000 calories per year—enough to
slough about fifteen extra pounds.

Children and teenagers can both be asked to use the
resources available in their schools and communities to

collect similar important information. Early in the program, it is wise to ask children to keep close records of what they eat and what they do. These can be the same records that are kept by adults, those shown on pages 14 and 196.

Using the data from these records, plans should be made for increasing activity. Adolescents should be encouraged to have as much social contact as possible and to use this contact as a means of building social skills. Because overweight adolescents are self-conscious and many have been the victims of ridicule by their classmates, they are often shy and inhibited. But all have a strong desire to make and to maintain friendships. The way to friendship is through progressively more varied activities. Good choices for activities are those that require intelligence, creativity, and interpersonal abilities, as well as those which build physical skill and dexterity.

A second important activity is self-care and grooming. Because overweight adolescents often feel that they do not compete successfully in the contest for good looks, many have a tendency toward carelessness in dress and grooming. Unfortunately, a careless appearance advertises self-disdain and invites social rejection. Therefore, efforts to improve personal tidiness are rarely wasted.

In addition, and most importantly, adolescents should be encouraged to increase their level of physical activity. Overweight people, in general, have a tendency to find energy-saving rather than energy-expending ways of using their bodies. Therefore, overweight children must begin to recondition themselves to stand rather than to sit, to move about rather than to stand, to walk rather than to ride, and to move quickly rather than slowly.

When the adolescent has identified weight as a problem worth concerted effort, parents can help by using the three tactics of social influence which have been described. The following table gives but a few illustrations:

	Moderate eating	Greater social activity	Better grooming	More physical activity
Example	Eat moderate meals	Engage in skill-building family activities	Attend to own personal appear-ance	Go for walks, begin physical activities
Prompt	Ask how much the adolescent plans to eat at the start of the meal	Arrange for other sitters to stay with younger sibs so that teenager can be with friends	Provide an adequate clothes budget	Provide easy access to sports facilities
Payoff	Warmly recognize moderate eating	Express interest in outside activities.	Notice improved appear-ance	Allow teen to keep bus or cab fare if he or she walks

Finally, because the normal relationship between parents and teenagers is fraught with difficulties, excessive involvement of the parent in the weight loss program may be a source of considerable strain. Therefore the teenager's participation in a self-chosen weight-loss program, whether through a clinic or a responsible weight-control organization such as "Weight Watchers," can often spell the difference between success and failure. While data on the subject are scarce, one study did show that obese teenagers who participated in a weight-loss group had half the number of personal problems as were reported by those who were nonparticipants.[15] Such participation has the advantages of offering professionally supervised program planning and group support from people who are clearly *not* involved in the resolution of identity growth crises at home.

How Spouses Can Help

Have you or your spouse gained weight since you married? Have you changed your eating habits in any important ways? Has your activity increased or decreased significantly? Has the role of food in your life altered significantly—that is, are you more or less likely to turn to food as a means of meeting a crisis? Many couples make these and more changes following their marriages. Read on, and meet some people who have had these experiences.

Tom and Roni have been married for six years. Before they were married, each held jobs in the plant, Tom as a relief foreman and Roni as a lab technician in the plastics department. Both were on the go much of the time and their meals were quick and light. The only times they had complete meals were at the family dinners they felt compelled to join. Tom played catcher on a semi-pro softball team and Roni was a figure skater. Both were Class A bowlers in a mixed Tuesday-night bowling league.

After they were married, Tom traded softball for night school and Roni gave up figure skating for pregnancy. They did continue to bowl on Tuesday nights but they cut out practice sessions to save money. Meals, which had been hasty affairs before marriage, later became important times. Roni felt that she had to compete with Tom's mother for culinary honors and she therefore learned to bake bread and pies and became a skilled gravy and sauce chef. Both paid closer attention to Roni's cuisine than to their swelling waistlines. Their problem: a sudden gain in the amount of food that they ate coupled with a drop in the level of their physical activity.

Al and Zena (known to their friends as the "A to Z" kids when they were courting) live next door to Tom and Roni. They were both plump when they were married. They have had four children and with each pregnancy Zena gained thirty pounds before delivery and lost only ten pounds afterward. Al is a solicitous husband who pays careful attention to Zena's every desire. He knows that she has a "sweet tooth" so he often surprises her with treats from her favorite bakery. Zena feels that Al is very sensitive and tries hard never to hurt his feelings. Therefore, even though she knows that the sweet treats are a problem for her, she heaves to when the bakery box arrives. For Al and Zena the problem is that each sees food as love: to give food is to express love and to eat food is to accept a loving offering.

Sid and Marcy who live farther down the block have a different problem. When all three families first moved onto the block they were quite friendly. But over the years, Sid and Marcy made their fights ever more public until the others began to shy away from them. Marcy's father had a drinking problem and she had a morbid dread and dislike of alcohol. As if to spite her, Sid began to drink and has now reached the point at which three doubles every evening are the minimum necessary "fuel for his burners." Sid has made clear to Marcy that he finds slender women attractive and heavy women gross. As if out of spite, Marcy has taken to eating up a storm whenever Sid takes a drink or does anything which she considers to be an insult. Sid uses alcohol as a weapon and Marcy uses food as a weapon. Their problem is that both work hard at destroying themselves instead of making a frontal assault on their relationship difficulties.

These are three common patterns—activity is allowed to decline while food intake rises, food is used as a means of expressing love, and eating is used as a form of expressing anger. There are many others. In each, food is permitted to become something which it is not. If food is used to placate the spouse, if it is used to pay for indulgence, if it is used instead of social contact, or if it is used as an arena in which to try unsuccessfully to resolve other marital stresses, eating can only cause more problems than it resolves.

Using the three tools of social influence—example, prompting, and paying off—these problem interactions can be reversed. It will naturally be easiest for Tom and Roni to set things straight in their home, but even Sid and Marcy can gain greatly from a few simple changes.

Set a Good Example

This means that each partner should eat the proper amounts of well-selected foods and shun overeating at mealtimes and problem treats between meals. It also means that each should get as much physical activity as is healthful and practical. This can be done in small ways by looking for opportunities to take extra steps instead of saving steps, and in larger ways by walking or planning some other activity every day.

Each partner should also set an example by acknowledging the positive things which the other does. There is strong evidence for the maxim that "Positive Input is Needed in Order to Change Relationships."[16] Negative exchanges help to fix behavior at its current level while positive exchanges make things better. For example, when Sid shouts "Stop that" at Marcy as she reaches for a second helping of dessert, he tells her that he will pay attention when she makes a mistake. "Stop that" shouters ignore positive behavior when it occurs and their negative communications tend to be the only attention which others receive. If when Marcy refuses a second helping of a tempting dish Sid said, "Marcy, that's great! I'm really impressed with what you're accomplishing!''—then Marcy would learn that she could earn Sid's attention through positive actions. Then and only then would she be in a position to make a strong run at achieving a major change. If Marcy wants Sid to treat her in this way, she must set an example by offering her praise when he curbs his drinking!

Prompt the Kind of Action That You Would Like to Have Happen

When one person decides to develop new eating patterns, that is an important change for the family. All behavioral patterns develop a certain momentum. Others in the family expect certain actions and respond to these actions in predictable ways. Many times family members inadvertently work to keep things as they have been; for example, they telegraph negative expectations: "Since you didn't get your way, Sid, I suppose you're going to hit the bottle again." With these words Marcy casts a role which Sid will find very difficult not to follow.

When new patterns emerge, readjustment is necessary. Even if the change is one which all in the family desire, others will have the tendency to keep acting as though the new behavior had not occurred. Therefore, each time that one person decides to make a change, it is very important that he or she announce what is planned and ask for the help that is desired. For example, Zena might say, "Al, I have been having some really bad feelings about myself and I have decided to start to lose weight. You could help me a lot by taking me to a show, asking me to go for a walk, or just sitting close to me to tell me that you care, and by helping me to keep sweets out of the house." That way Al can hear Zena's message loud and clear and it will be his choice whether to help or to hinder her efforts.

Marcy found from her self-monitoring chart that her problem eating tended to occur at three different times:

while she prepared meals, when she ate alone because Sid stayed late at the store, and when she was angry. Sid used the Keep Track chart to get a fix on his drinking. He found that he downed half of his liquor before dinner every night and the other half when he felt alone and annoyed later in the evening.

When they compared notes, Sid and Marcy found that they could make some pleasant changes. Marcy realized she felt rejected when Sid came home in the evening, took his drink into the living room, and read the paper while she finished dinner. She asked Sid to keep her company and even to pitch in as one way to help her overcome her late-afternoon depressions. For his part, Sid liked this early-evening contact and he was able to lessen his before-dinner drinking. Marcy asked Sid please to let her know at least a day in advance when he planned to stay late at the store so that she could prepare her dinner ahead of time and have only the proper portions ready. That way she avoided cooking for two and having extra food readily available when she felt lonely. Sid and Marcy also agreed to spend at least an hour together every evening after dinner. Whether they just talked, played cards, read, or watched television together, each felt a kind of closeness during this time. It cut down Marcy's feelings of anger and Sid's feelings of isolation. Each thus prompted the other to make a change that could go far toward creating a positive climate, as well as breaking early links in the problem-eating chain.

There are hundreds of other prompts which may be useful. One wife asks her husband to serve her portions of food, knowing that he will not make the mistake of giving her a little extra. Another wife asks for her husband's company while she cleans up after dinner, knowing that when he is with her she will be able to resist the temptation to eat table scraps. Still another wife asks her husband to phone her at exactly 12:30 every day: she begins her lunch at about ten past twelve and uses his call as a signal to leave the kitchen and get started with her afternoon activities. A husband asks his wife to make lunch for him so that he can avoid the temptations of going past the cafeteria food displays, while another husband prompts his wife to have apples instead of peanuts available for snacks.

To find the kind of prompts that will help you, look over your eating record carefully and identify the times when eating is a problem.

Discuss these times with your partner and work together on a suggestion list which will serve as his or her prompts for your new eating routine.

Pay Off the Behaviors Which You Wish to Have Continued

There are two common problems in the payoff department. First, we all have a tendency to pay more attention to negative behavior than to positive. We tend to react to negatives as if they were intentional wounds while we respond to positives as though they were our perfect right. In order to set this situation straight, considerable attention must be paid to offering strong and unambiguous payoffs for constructive behaviors.

The second problem in managing payoff properly is that we all have an inclination to act inconsistently. Inconsistency can lead to confusing double messages. For example, after Zena asked Al to find ways other than food gifts to express affection, he did make an effort to be inventive. After a time, however, he passed a shop with marzipan fruits in the window. He knew that Zena had a passion for marzipan, so he decided to bring home a real surprise—"to show what a good job he thought she was doing." As soon as Zena saw the candy, she felt two very strong conflicting emotions: she did love marzipan, but she knew how terrible she would feel if she gave in to temptation. If she smiled warmly and accepted the candy, in effect she would have told Al to disregard her earlier prompt and go back to the candy-as-usual routine. If she accepted the candy, she would undermine her own good efforts. What she had to do is:

1. Relate to the underlying positive feeling in the offer;
2. And then consistently refuse.
3. Suggest a nonfood alternative.

Zena might say, "Al, I know that you want to do something special for me and you know that marzipan used to be my passion. But now it is really important for me to get myself under good control and I'd love it if you would offer to take me to the movies instead of buying sweets when you want to tell me that you care." That way Al knows that Zena has heard the important message—he loves her—but he also knows the way in which he can help her best. Zena is then faced with the difficult task of setting the marzipan aside and not taking even a single taste of this or any future treat.

Very often painful choices must be made. In the long run, everyone's interests are best served when alternatives to food are sought and used as a means of expressing affection, coping with strong emotions, relieving boredom, and the like. As Zena begins to feel better about herself, she will have much more to offer Al and he will then be richly rewarded for his efforts to help her succeed. Therefore, while it may be difficult, *absolute consistency* is required in paying off others for helpful changes, whatever they may be.

In a Nutshell

Some important points have been made in this chapter. First, it was pointed out, through a review of the scientific literature of the past four decades, that obesity is a family affair. Whether or not families create problems of overweight in their members, families certainly help to maintain overeating and inactivity. By the same

token, families can be invaluable resources in meeting
the challenge of developing better eating and activity
patterns. Once the overeater/underexerciser has reached
the decision that change is needed—and it must be his or
her personal decision—help from other family members
can be carefully planned using the three techniques of
social influence. The steps are simple:

1. Working from your Self-Monitoring Chart, identify
   times when problem eating occurs and times when
   physical activity can be expanded;
2. For each time decide:
   a. Which family member will set what good example?
   b. Which family member will offer which prompts? By
      word? And/or by action?
   c. And finally, which family member will offer what
      kind of payoff?

Plans should be made by all members of the family
working as a team. The plans should be simple in order
to be realistic. They must call for positive interactions
only—*no negative prompts, no negative payoff*. And
they must include an opportunity for each person to
keep track of what he or she does pursuant to the plan.

If Dad and Jenny agree that Jenny should walk to
school each day, and that Dad will walk with her and
take the bus from her school to his office, then Dad
should keep track of the days on which he sets this good
example. If Al agrees to serve Zena's portions and to
keep the serving dishes near the stove rather than on the
table so that Zena is not tempted to take seconds, then
he should keep track of the times that he remembers to
do so. Finally, if Sid agrees to spend fifteen minutes
with Marcy in the kitchen each evening, as a way of
paying her off for curbing her urge to eat during the late
afternoon, then he, too, should keep track of his efforts. The form which can be used for these records is
illustrated in Figure 13.1.

None of these steps has to be complex. For example,
it was found that one woman consumed 1,251 calories
in three night-eating bouts when she was alone, and 185

calories in three other bouts when her husband was present.[17] Therefore, the mere presence of a family member can act as a prompt for prudent food selection and portion control.

FIGURE 13.1

A Chart for Keeping Track of How Some
Family Members Help Others

Who?
Will set what Example?
Will offer which Prompts?
Will Pay Off good behaviors in what way?

It was done the following times on the following days:

	MONDAY	TUESDAY	WEDNESDAY	THURSDAY	FRIDAY	SATURDAY	SUNDAY
Example							
Prompt							
Pay Off							

CHAPTER 14

Working Down an Appetite While Working Spirits Up

THERE WAS A time when the sidewalks of Everytown, U.S.A., were crowded: now strollers are the exception and not the rule. Our ballfields were once jammed with eager sportsmen of all ages: now most of us spend our Sundays as TV jocks and the parks are the province of "health nuts" and the young. We used to sharpen our own pencils, chop ice for our own martinis, and open our own cans by hand: now these and dozens of other minor jobs have become the work of our electronic slaves. We have refined the art of doing nothing to such a point that we even have machines to rub our backs when they ache from inactivity. In short, we will spare no expense and apply the heights of our ingenuity to any task that will allow us to push a button rather than move an arm, to sit instead of stand, or to ride rather than walk. We have reached that unhappy moment when no task is too slight to warrant calling upon a machine to do the job for us, and no trip too short to hold us back from climbing into the family car.

The result of this energy-sparing way of life is serious. We have become a nation of heavy-limbed, stiff-jointed armchair dwellers. As a result, our bellies have broadened and our stamina has waned.

I'm Heavy Already: What Good Can Activity Do Me Now?

It is not at all unusual to read statements like the following: "Overweight? Forget exercise. You'd have to climb to the top of the Empire State Building three times in a row to lose one single pound," or "If you're trying to walk your weight off, forget it! You have to walk from dawn to dusk to get rid of one pound of fat."

While some authorities question the role of activity in weight control, the Food and Nutrition Board of the National Research Council clearly recognizes its importance. In its Recommended Dietary Allowances, *the* authoritative statement of minimum nutritional needs, the Council considered activity to be the "dominant factor leading to variability in energy needs."[1] Specifically, the Council recommends that men and women who engage in moderate activity consume 300 more calories per day than those whose activity is light, and that those who engage in heavy activity take in 600 to 900 calories more to meet their extra energy needs. It therefore stands to reason that anyone who holds caloric intake constant and increases the level of activity would have to burn fat stores to fuel this extra effort.

Let's look at what happens with a 125-pound woman and a 150-pound man. The sleeping woman burns approximately 1.0 calories per minute and the man 1.1. Sitting or standing, the woman burns up to 2.0 calories, the man up to 2.5. Walking slowly on a level surface, the woman burns up to 3.9 calories per minute, the man up to 4.9. Walking briskly on a level surface accounts for up to 5.9 calories per minute for women and 7.4 calories for men. And walking up a hill while carrying a load can account for 10.0 and 12.0 calories per minute for a woman and man respectively. In other words, vigorous activity requires over five times the calories burned while sitting still.

What does this mean for Joe and Jane who think about activity as a way of trying to burn off their extra fat? Assuming that they each weigh 150 pounds, they would have to spend about seventeen minutes walking or four minutes running to burn up the calories in an extra banana. Getting rid of the extra calories in a donut would require about twenty-nine minutes of walking or eight minutes of running. An ice cream soda is worth a forty-nine-minute walk or a thirteen-minute run. And a generous helping of strawberry shortcake would keep them on the sidewalk for seventy-seven minutes or on the track for twenty-one.[2]

All of this seems like a large effort for a small reward, but we get a different picture when we take a closer look. Our 150-pounder burns about 5.2 calories per minute while walking. If he or she goes for a thirty-minute stroll this would burn up about 150 calories. If the walk were taken five days each week for a year, and *if food intake stayed the same* throughout the year, 39,150 extra calories would be burned or enough to shed over eleven pounds in twelve months, twenty-two pounds in two years. What is more, if Joe or Jane weighed more than 150 pounds, their rewards would be even greater because it takes greater energy to move heavier bodies through space. For example, a small, lean man running a mile in about ten minutes will use 121 calories, but a 220-pound man running the same mile will burn 219 calories in the same amount of time.[3] Therefore the more you work, the longer you spend at it, and the heavier you are, the more calories you will burn for the effort.

Finally, as an added bonus, it is important to note that the weight-related benefit of exercise extends long after the exerciser sits down to rest. In one controlled experiment, resting metabolism four hours after a vigorous workout was from 7.5 to 28 percent *higher* than it was at the same time on days when no exercise took place.[4] That means that hours after activity ends, our bodies still burn extra fat. Clearly, then, an increase in activity can be of considerable value in using up unwanted calories.

The value of increased activity goes far beyond its impact upon weight. It can improve the health of the heart and circulatory system in several different ways, not the least of which is by preventing the buildup of extra cholesterol in the bloodstream and by cutting down the amount of fat that's already there.[5] It can also improve your state of mind in six important ways; even a small increase in the amount of physical activity can help to:

1. Reduce the level of tension and stresses which you experience;
2. Help you to rest more comfortably and to sleep better;
3. Help to improve your concentration and enthusiasm for work and play;
4. Help to improve your mood;
5. Help to reduce your appetite; and
6. Help to improve your self-confidence.[6]

Increased activity can help to reduce tension because tension is, at its root, a physical experience. As you learned in Chapter 11, helping muscles to relax, the cues that trigger the psychological experience of stress can be minimized. When you feel less tension, you are likely to find relaxation easier and sleep deeper and more satisfying. Feeling better rested, you are almost certain to find it easier to concentrate on your work and to meet the challenges of everyday living. This, in turn, can give rise to more positive experiences in work and play, both of which logically help you to feel positive as well. Then your lowered tension, greater rest, concentration, enthusiasm, and improved mood all combine to help *reduce your urge to eat.* Instead of working *up* an appetite, research has clearly shown that *light to moderate activity works appetite down.*[7] Repeat: *Research has shown that food intake decreases when work load moves from light to moderate.*

Moderate increases in activity appear to cut the urge

to eat and help to burn stored fat in the bargain. With all of these systems "go," it is small wonder that increased activity can help you to feel better about yourself and more confident in the future.

Increased activity feeds into improved self-esteem in two other ways. First, when you do something active you are doing something for all the world to see. You know, and others can know too, that you have taken action to help yourself. This is different from those dozens of good decisions that you make not to eat this or that: they are nonactions, they can't be seen. They are very important decisions but they do not offer you the same opportunity to stand up and be counted as does taking the bold step into increased activity.

Second, increased activity has a very important symbolic value. When you follow through on your commitment to yourself in this specific way, you know that you have finished a job well done. This can go far toward building your motivation to meet other challenges throughout the week. Activity, then, seems to be as good for your spirit as for your body, and it is clear that you can gain a lifetime of benefit from a little extra effort every day.

A Caution

An increase in activity should not be undertaken without specific medical approval by anyone who has suffered any cardiovascular stress, including hypertension and heart attacks. Those who have diabetes, electrolyte imbalances, anemia, varicose veins, and various other medical problems must also plan any activity with great care.[8]

If you are very much overweight or very much out of shape, a rapid increase in activity could lead to joint problems or other forms of physical stress. Therefore, it is important to rule out these or other kinds of potential dangers (rare though they may be) by *consulting with your doctor before you start to move about.*

Activity "Won'ts"

Several assumptions lead people to steer clear of healthful physical activity. We have already knocked out the excuse that activity has to be avoided for fear of working up an appetite. But "committed passives" have many other lines of defense against becoming active. For example, many people think that "physical activity" means "vigorous exercise" of the smelly sweatsuit variety. This is not necessarily the case! Physical activity means any effort to move your body around more than is your normal pattern. You can be physically active without getting out of breath, without getting overheated, and without changing from your everyday street clothes. In fact, the kind of exercise for which you do suit up may not suit you at all. It usually implies toe touching and knee bending, exercises which can be useful but which are often so uncomfortable that they are rarely pursued long enough to be of benefit.

Another excuse offered by people who won't increase their activity is that exercise is dull. Here, we run into semantics again. Perhaps stretching the same muscle for count after count is dull. Perhaps going through the same routine won't hold your interest. The fact is, though, that there are dozens of activities that can be useful to you, and you certainly can vary them to hold your interest every single day.

Some people won't exercise because they do not want to call public attention to themselves. But many activities can be done in the privacy of your own home and others can be done in unobtrusive ways in public places. For example, climbing stairs in your own home or office several extra times a day can be very useful.

Another activity "won't" stems from the belief that any useful program requires too much planning or too many people. Sure, if baseball is your number, you need seventeen others to help you out, or if jai alai is your choice, you'll have to find a court. But you can also choose from numerous solo ventures (e.g., swimming, bicycling, ice skating, rope jumping, or hitting a tennis ball against a wall) and activities that require neither companions nor equipment, such as walking, jogging, and climbing stairs.

Finally, the most basic unrealized excuse for avoiding exercise is simply that it involves change. Increasing activity means using muscles that may have been in mothballs for years, and it means getting in touch with your body in ways that you may not have experienced before. Above all, it means that you must develop some new attitudes and this may be the most difficult change of all.

Activity Choices

Once you have overcome your excuses for not becoming more active, you are faced with the challenge of deciding what to do. As a general rule:

1. You want to change your lifestyle in as many small and large ways as possible to
2. Increase the amount of energy that you spend in doing what you do all day long.

To do this you will have to:

1. Find ways to use more energy in your everyday activities; and
2. Choose new activities to build onto the things that you do.

At home, if you normally sit while talking on the telephone, try standing. If you normally ask others to bring the plates to you so you can wash the dishes, get the dishes yourself. If you normally sit and do nothing after dinner, plan a twenty-minute stroll. If you normally leave the heavy cleaning to someone else, think about doing more of it yourself. If you clean the basement and the garage once each year, think about bringing them up to snuff more often. In other words, change your daily routine so that during the time that you are at home your body is much more active.

You can also change your style on the job. If you normally ride the bus to work, try boarding the bus a stop or two farther from your home and then plan to get off a stop or two before your office. If you drive to work and park next door, park several blocks away instead. If you normally use the elevator in the building, think about using the stairs instead. If you normally sit at your desk or in the staff cafeteria for breaks, think about using the time to walk through the halls around the building, or walk to a more distant place to eat. If you eat lunch in the staff cafeteria, try walking several blocks to a sandwich shop instead. If you rely upon others to bring work to you, see if you can't find ways to fetch the supplies yourself. Again the watch word is: *do as much as you can yourself, relying as little as possible on others.*

The caloric differentials for each one of these small changes are not large, although they all can add up to a sizable energy expenditure over time. For example, if you stand instead of sitting you burn 1.5 instead of 1.3 calories per minute. If you walk instead of stand, your caloric use jumps from 1.5 to 3.1 per minute. If you walk downstairs instead of riding the elevator, you use 7.1 calories per minute instead of 1.5. And if you walk upstairs, it's 10.0 per minute instead of 1.5. Moreover, you can raise the ante 10 percent for each fifteen pounds that you weigh above 150, so that a 225-pound man burns 15 calories to the 150-pounder's 10 calories for each minute of stair climbing, or 150 in ten minutes as against the thin man's 100.[9] Because the increases in energy expenditure are cumulative—that is, every little bit counts—you do not have to exert yourself all at once. For instance, the 225-pounder who normally makes four trips each day up and down five stories in an elevator can use up a significant amount of energy by using the stairs instead as often as possible.

Beyond these frequent and small increases in physical activity, it is wise to plan a once-a-day larger activity as well. You might plan a walk each day. Choose an amount of time that you would like to spend and plan a gradual increase in the distance you travel during this time. That way, you will build up your stamina and, naturally, the farther you go per unit of time, the more energy you will spend in the effort. Many people find a twenty-minute walk both pleasurable and beneficial.

You can also choose a sport. You may follow your sport once or more each week, and you may choose more than one sport in any week. Rowing, skating, and cycling slowly can take care of 5 calories per minute, while doing any of them at a faster clip can be worth up to 15. Ping-Pong is worth 5 to 7 calories per minute, tennis 7 to 11, and dancing 5 to 8. Running a mile in twelve minutes is a 120-calorie effort, while running two miles in the same time burns twice the energy. And once again, the more you weigh, the greater will be your caloric loss.[10]

In working out a plan for personal activity, it is a good idea to follow five specific rules, after having your doctor's okay:

1. Choose an activity that is natural for you, not one which you think that you "should" select.
2. Plan specific activity times for every single day.
3. Make activity a daily rather than a sometime commitment.
4. If you can, find someone to join in your activities, but always be prepared to go it alone.
5. Start small, work your way up.

Choosing to do things that come naturally is important because you are obviously less likely to follow through on programs which "put you out of joint." Planning to follow through on your activity at specific times each day will increase the chance that the activity gets done. You do not have to choose the same time every day. For example, after work on weekdays and early morning on the weekends might be one person's choice, while another might take the early mornings during the week and afternoons on weekends. Just as you individualize the choice of which activity you will pursue, so, too, should you individualize when you plan to follow through.

You also have to make the decision to follow through with an activity that can be done every single day. If you allow the weather to be a factor, you'll risk breaking the activity habit. If you depend upon others to fire you up, their unavailability can stand in your way. Therefore, just as you have backup plans for each step in breaking your eating chain, have backup plans for foul weather and solo days. For example, if you walk/jog for twenty minutes a day, be ready with a stair climb in bad weather. If you plan a tennis game, be ready for a brisk walk around the park if your partner fails to appear.

Now that you know the essentials, the next move is yours. Make that move now! The longer you wait, the less likely it is that you'll act. Use the chart in Figure 14.1 to plan your program. And then follow through with your plans to the best of your ability. Your rewards will be higher spirits, fewer urges to eat, and a gradual reduction in your excess weight.

IN A NUTSHELL

Many people believe that activity builds appetite. The fact is, however, that increased activity can *lower* your urge to eat. It can also improve your spirits and your health. To become more active you must overcome the tendency to equate activity with work. You can increase your activity by adding energy to the things that you normally do every day. You can also increase your activity by planning some kind of mild or moderate exercise for a short time every day. By changing your lifestyle to include more use of energy, you can do yourself inestimable good.

FIGURE 14.1

My Activity Planner

Day	Exactly what time will I begin and end?	What's my first-choice activity?	What's my backup if the weather is bad or I'm alone?
Monday			
Tuesday			
Wednesday			
Thursday			
Friday			
Saturday			
Sunday			

CHAPTER 15

Heading Off Binges at the Pass

BINGE EATING POSES the same threat to the person seeking weight control that tornadoes do to the plains dweller, that typhoons do to the South Sea islander, and that blizzards do to the people of the Arctic: they threaten to destroy a lifetime of effort. But binges, unlike forces of nature, are controllable, psychologically motivated events. And even though binges might not be prevented, some precautions can help to lessen their ravages.

Binges mean different things to different people. Some regard a slight extra indulgence as a binge, but others do not feel they have binged unless they have eaten madly for hours or even days. Binge eating usually begins with a combination of moods, such as boredom and anger. Binges start small and build up rapidly, and they are more likely to occur on days when regular meals have been skipped. Members of Weight Watchers classes were asked to describe the binges they experienced before becoming members. One person in eight reported binging on days when they had eaten all three meals, one in four reported binging on days when they had skipped breakfast, and three out of five of those who skipped breakfast and lunch reported binging as a major problem. Therefore, negative moods and omitted meals can set the stage for binging.

Members of Weight Watchers classes also reported that binges tended to begin at night, although they might extend into the following day; that binging almost always took place at home; that they almost always hid binge eating from others; that binges often began with small or moderate amounts of a preferred food, but then went on to include larger amounts of almost anything; and that they rarely knew how much they ate either during or after a binge. These observations have helped me to formulate a five-step program for binge control:

1. When you feel the desire to eat a between-meal snack, try distraction first by turning to something other than food.
2. After you experience the urge to eat, wait at least ten minutes to begin eating.
3. When you do eat, choose a food that is not on your "much preferred" list.
4. Take the smallest possible quantity of the food that you eat. If you go back for more, again take the smallest possible helping.
5. Consider anything that you have eaten to be water over the dam. Don't dwell on it. Begin immediately to follow your original eating plan.

Distraction can help to break your preoccupation with eating. You can distract yourself by making a change in your environment and your activity. If you are sitting in the living room and the urge to eat strikes, move to the basement, the bedroom, or the backyard— go anyplace where you will not be in contact with food. If you are watching TV when the urge to eat strikes, turn the TV off and play your favorite album. If you are reading, try TV. If you are cleaning, turn to a hobby.

Do anything that will change your environment and occupy your mind. In changing both environment and activity, you take into account that your urge to eat is a response to your present situation: *Change the situation and you can limit the urge to eat*.

As the impulse to binge begins to develop, you may become aware of a powerful obsession about eating in general or about the taste or texture of certain foods. For example, Jody traced her binge impulse to frustration at work, where she was often asked to do more than could reasonably be expected in the time allowed, besides having to wait sometimes four or five weeks for what were to have been weekly paychecks. Following peaks in this frustration, she would begin to think about food as she drove home, with the thoughts growing more and more compelling with each passing mile. By the time she was halfway home, she could think of nothing but the taste and texture of her favorite candy bars; and once she reached that level of obsession, she was all but certain to find the nearest convenience food store where she could buy a dozen candy bars "for a friend's party," as she told the clerk. She then ate them one after another while she finished her journey, dropping the wrappers in a trashcan at a gas station so that all of the immediate outward signs of her binge would go undetected.

Because Jody was aware that her binge eating was often triggered by frustration, she knew when she should be on guard. She also knew that several passing thoughts about candy were likely to lead to total immersion in fantasies of candy-bar land. She could use this information to cue herself to a technique called "thought stopping," and thus free herself before a full-blown obsession took hold.

Thought stopping is a technique first described by Dr. Joseph Cautela of Boston College University.[1] Quite simply, it involves learning to stop one thought by starting another, rather than simply trying to make the negative thought disappear. (Try *not* thinking about camels for the next 60 seconds if you think that you can erase a

thought without replacing it.) You can quickly teach
yourself this technique by following these four steps:

1. Identify situations in which you are likely to feel a strong
   impulse to binge eat.
2. Identify the early stages of your overeating obsession;
   for instance, think about the smell, appearance, taste, or
   texture of some favorite food, or think about your
   pleasure in biting and swallowing large quantities of
   foods.
3. Take a mental inventory of the things that please you
   most in life, whether experienced or imagined.
4. Then learn to wipe your mental slate clean, getting rid of
   the binge-eating picture by replacing it with highly
   valued alternative pictures.

For example, Jody's happiest memories of her college
days were those of winning freestyle swimming races in
intercollegiate competition. She could recall the sting of
the water at the instant of her initial dive, could feel her
body part the water as the thrust propelled her swiftly
just an inch or two below its surface, and then could
recall the sensation in her shoulders as each stroke
steadily pulled water from the front and pushed it
behind to move her rapidly ahead. She loved that feeling, and the sensation in her lungs as she took rapid,
shallow breaths, the sound of the bubbles as her head
turned in the water, and the look of the tile pattern on
the stripes marking lane boundaries on the bottom of
the pool. And, of course, she could describe with excitement her joy at each smooth, porpoise-like turn at the
end of each lap, and the exhilaration she felt when she
reached the finish line first. For her then, thoughts of all
of the strong sensations of swimming to victory would
easily conquer annoying visions of forbidden foods.

You should make an inventory of your happier images, things that you may already have experienced or
would like to experience. They can involve seeing yourself in beautiful places, doing wonderful things, or interacting with fascinating people. You should file away
in the back of your mind at least three such images, and

you should be ready to pull the file and summon up its rich detail using all your senses: sight, touch, smell, hearing—but not taste. The more prized and detailed the image, the more powerful it will be in purging your urge to binge.

Thought stopping will nearly always provide enough distraction so that you can wait at least ten minutes before bringing food to mouth. The ten-minute wait will give you time to think. It can help to break the grip of your preoccupation with food, giving you an opportunity to become interested in other things. Waiting the ten minutes can also give you proof that you are still in control. This renewed self-confidence can help you to limit your eating at this time. Use a kitchen timer that sounds a bell to time the ten-minute interval. When the bell rings, if you have it in you to wait ten minutes more, set the timer and see what you can do.

Choosing a nonpreferred food is a very important link in this urge-control chain. Research has shown that while the obese are not more sensitive to the taste of food than are the lean,[2] many overweight people do have difficulty in limiting the foods they prefer.[3] Because your resistance is low when you are set to binge, you may experience a tendency to eat far too much of your favorite foods. Moreover, if you eat your favorite foods at these times, you are, in effect, rewarding yourself for allowing your eating to get out of hand.

Make a list of the foods that you particularly like as snack foods (using the spaces below), and a second list of nonpreferred foods that are generally on hand. For example, you might like cookies, nuts, and chocolate as snacks; they would go on your "Preferred: To Be Avoided" list. On the other hand, your refrigerator could always be stocked with carrots, celery, radishes, or pepper strips; they can be added to your "I Don't Like These As Well So They're Okay" list.

Preferred: To Be Avoided	I Don't Like These As Well So They're Okay
1. _____	1. _____
2. _____	2. _____
3. _____	3. _____
4. _____	4. _____

Many dieters take an all-or-nothing approach to their food management. As suggested in Chapter 3, they are "dichotomous thinkers." It has been shown, for example, that when dieters in a research setting were given an opportunity to have a snack, those who thought they had broken their diets ate more than those who believed they had eaten only what they should. In actual truth, both had eaten exactly the same amount before they had been given a chance to snack. The message is this:

> DO ALL YOU CAN TO MAKE CERTAIN
> THAT EVERY TIME YOU EAT
> YOU HAVE GIVEN YOURSELF AN OPPORTUNITY
> TO DRAW THE FINAL LINE.

If you plan to eat a slice of bread and know that you should eat only one slice, take it, close the package, return it to its proper place, and go to the table where you will sit and eat it. Go back, if you must, to take a second slice, but repeat the same routine. If you take the package to the table with you, you are likely to eat "automatically," you will lose track of how much you eat, and you will not stop yourself before the damage is done.

Finally, after you have started to snack and you realize that you are deviating from your eating plan, it is essential that you give yourself constructive messages. Many binge eaters tell themselves that they have done a "terrible thing" and have proven that they have "no willpower." These are self-indulgent statements that merely set the stage for further problem eating. Instead, you should treat management of your urge to eat as a challenge. Ask yourself the question, "How can I keep my eating within bounds?" instead of making self-derogatory statements. Because your thoughts guide your actions, directing your thoughts constructively can help you to keep your actions in check.

If you do binge, it is essential to bear in mind that every binge comes to an end. Some end sooner than others, but no one ever goes on eating forever! As soon as the binge ends, you must turn your attention to the next events in your life. Never, never allow yourself to dwell on the binge. If you must think about it at all, think what you can do in the future to make binging less likely to occur or to be weaker if it does occur. To keep your thoughts in this constructive vein, take a pencil and paper and list the binge-control actions that you think would be helpful in the future. Probably the worst thing that you can do is to punish yourself for yesterday's binge, because the guilt it creates is likely to do little more than bring on another binge tomorrow.

The second most fatal after-binging mistake you can make is to skip meals to make up for the previous excess. All this does is create a "caloric debt" or a belief that you owe yourself something for having been so prudent as to omit some eating opportunities. It also builds hunger that you are most likely to satisfy with between-meal eating; and, as you well know, these are the times that you are most likely to eat too much of the wrong kinds of food.

In a Nutshell

Managing binge eating begins with controlling your moods and planning your meals wisely. Also, you should have a strategy ready that will allow you to break the chain of binge eating early and often, so that you have the greatest possible number of opportunities to keep your eating within reasonable bounds. Panic is the greatest single threat to the binge eater. Preplanning and a realization that binging only means that the first set of limits was ineffective, so a second line of defense is needed, can help both to control the panic and to contain the damage that binges can do. Above all, when binging slows down your weight-control efforts, take the binge in your stride and continue with your self-management program at the earliest possible moment. Binging does not create disaster; overreaction to binges is the major villain.

CHAPTER 16

Planning What to Eat

UP TO THIS point, you have been taught how to manage your urge to eat. Now it is time to talk about what to eat.

Weight is maintained when the body takes in just enough energy in the form of food to keep its vital processes going and its muscles active. Weight is gained when more energy is taken in than is needed for these two purposes, and weight is lost when energy consumption falls below energy need. In other words, *weight is a simple product of supply and demand*. When the supply and demand of energy are in balance, weight is maintained. When supply exceeds demand weight is gained, and when demand is greater than supply weight is lost.

When we take in more energy than we need at the moment, our bodies burn what is required and store most of the rest. Later, if energy demands become greater than outside energy supply, our bodies turn to their stores and burn some of this supply. When we gain weight we store energy against future needs, and when we lose weight we literally burn up some of this supply.

When we store extra energy for future needs, we do to ourselves the same thing that we do to our cars when we put gas in the tank. The average gas tank holds enough fuel to allow the car to cruise from 200 to 400 miles between filling stations. If the car's gas tank were enlarged so that it could hold 200 gallons instead of 20 gallons, it would have a greater cruising range. But 20 gallons of gasoline weighs under 200 pounds and 200 gallons weighs close to 2,000 pounds. To handle that added weight the car would have to be built much more sturdily, it would have to lose considerable maneuverability, and it would get fewer miles to the gallon. The same is true for humans. If we normally store enough energy for five or six days of life, but add to our supplies enough for fifty or sixty days, we strain our body structures, we curtail our mobility, and we get sharply reduced mileage from the food that we consume.

The energy balance equation is universal but it does not apply with equal efficiency to all people. Some overweight people eat more than some of the lean, as found when their behavior is observed in public eating places.[1] But many others eat as little or even less than the lean, with the major difference being not how much energy goes in, but how much energy goes out in the form of physical activity.[2] The balance between intake, output, and fat storage is not one of a simple two-plus-two-equals-four mathematics. Somewhere in the process, some people seem able to "waste" some calories: they eat a lot, do little, and still don't gain very much weight. Other people are very efficient and for them every calorie counts. For all, however, the basic weight-control formula is the same: cut intake relative to output to lose weight, and reverse the process to put weight on.

Our bodies store energy in three forms. Some energy is stored as *carbohydrates* (actually glycogen and sugar) in the bloodstream, muscles, and liver. This energy supply is very important because it is the immediately available fuel for the organs and it sustains life. A feeling of faintness can result when this supply falls below the necessary life-supporting level. Therefore, the body works hard to keep an adequate supply of glycogen or blood sugar at all times.

Energy is also stored as *protein*, which is the building block of muscles and organs. The conversion of protein to energy could seriously weaken the body because tissue loss from any of its muscles, the heart, brain, and liver, or other organs can impair its ability to survive. Moreover, protein is a poor source of fuel. Protein supplies only 4 calories of energy per gram. (A calorie is the amount of heat—i.e., energy—needed to heat one gram of water, one degree centigrade.) And because protein is about 80 percent water, one pound of it would net only 450 calories or about one-sixth of the daily energy need of a typical young man. Because the body seems to have an inner wisdom, it turns to protein as an energy supply only after it has exhausted the energy that has been stored as fat.

Fat is the best of the body's energy supplies. It yields 9 calories per gram and, because fat is only 15 percent fluid, *one pound of fat yields 3,500 calories*. This is the critical number for all weight losers because, within small variations, the average man or woman who takes in an extra 3,500 calories—over a period of hours, days, or weeks—gains close to one pound of fat while the person who takes in 3,500 calories less than he or she burns—again over a period of hours, days, or weeks—will lose one pound of fat, give or take a little.

We can see the importance to reducers of the number 3,500 in the following illustration taken from the medical literature. Mrs. "Green" is a thirty-year old housewife who is five feet four inches tall. She weighs 225 pounds. We can assume for the purpose of this illustration that she normally needs 2,600 calories to keep her vital life-sustaining processes going and to supply the energy which she needs to go on about her business. If she cuts her daily food intake to approximately 1,200 calories, and if she maintains her usual level of activity, she would draw upon her energy reserves for 1,400 calories daily. In two days this would mean that she would burn up 2,800 calories' worth of fat tissues, in three days 4,200 calories' worth, and so on. Every day that she registers a 1,400-calorie deficit she could lose 0.4 pounds of fat, although this loss will not register on the scale every day. If her goal weight is 125 pounds she has 100 pounds to lose, losing 0.4 pounds per day, it should take her 250 days to reach her goal weight.[3]

Because the body can do nothing with extra energy other than to store it, taking in even a few extra calories every day can lead to a large aggregate weight gain. For example, eating one small extra cookie or one large extra apple per day (70 calories) would lead to the gain of an extra pound of fat every seven weeks, or between seven and eight pounds per year. Carried over a period of four or five years, this very small indulgence can lead to a very significant weight problem. Fortunately, however, the same pattern works in reverse. Eliminating one cookie or one extra fruit from your daily diet can lead to a very satisfying weight loss at year's end.

Because most of us are impatient, we are dissatisfied with the prospect of taking 250 days to achieve any goal, even one as important as losing 100 pounds. Some people try to speed up the process by using mechanical reducing aids. Others take pills with or without their doctor's prescription. Still others try to eat as little as possible, often without medical supervision.

There are three problems with all of these schemes. First, it is often either unhealthy or impossibly uncomfortable to follow them for very long. Second, during the process of losing weight no new constructive habits are learned. Therefore, maintaining the loss of weight is all but impossible. Indeed, research done on many of the tested quick-loss schemes (and most have not been researched) nearly always shows that weight lost in a hurry is regained just about as fast. This sets the stage for the third problem with rapid weight loss: if it leads to quick regains it can be quite bad for your health.

The chief of the Heart Disease Control Program of the United States Public Health Service has suggested that the "yo-yo" pattern of weight loss and gain may be worse for your health than just staying as overweight as you were in the first place.[4] He pointed out, for example, that (1) laboratory animals that are allowed to stay thin live longer than those that are allowed overeat, underexercise, and therefore become fat; but (2) that those staying fat lived longer than those whose weight fluctuated between thinness and fatness. He also pointed out that cholesterol or fat deposits build up in the bloodstream while weight is being gained, and that there is no evidence that these deposits are lost when excess pounds are shed. Crushed self-esteem and the very real possibility of major problems in blood chemistry are just two of the unwelcome consequences of attempts to lose too quickly and too easily. Therefore, you will do well to pass by those wonder diets, devices, and drugs that may have been promoted by people who claim to have "discovered nature's long-buried secret."

What you need instead is a program that will lead to the loss of from one to two pounds per week, unless you are very much overweight and under a doctor's care.[5] Any program that brings you down too quickly is likely to bump you back up just as fast, and you'll be much the worse for wear.

Diets of from 1,100 to 1,400 calories per day for women, and of 1,500 to 1,800 calories per day for men, are likely to offer the opportunity for just such a gradual loss of weight. The lower end of the calorie range would be best for you if you are less active or are in the lower weight range for your sex and height, and you will need the higher end of the range if you are more active than most and if you are on the husky side compared to your peers.

The diet that you choose must have these four important characteristics beyond offering gradual loss of weight:

1. It must provide all of your minimum daily food requirements;
2. It must give you enough to eat so that you are not faced with constant hunger;
3. It must give you enough variety every day so that your desire for different tastes and textures is satisfied; and
4. Following the weight-loss program must provide you with an education for lifelong changes in what you eat.

If the program that you choose does not meet your body's daily nutritional needs, you will run the risk of suffering one of several serious nutritional inadequacies that could seriously impair your health. This will cause true hunger and malnutrition. If you eat so little that you are always hungry, you are likely to experience a tormented existence and quickly give up your diet. Your appetite will never rest. If you eat the same few foods day after day, the monotony will cause you to stray from your program. Again, your appetite will rear its nasty head. And if the diet that you follow is eccentric because it gives you little choice or requires you to eat foods that are not normally available, you will have little chance of following the program in the years after your weight goal has been reached.

To find a food plan that meets these requirements—gradual loss, nutritional balance, prevention of hunger, satisfaction to your appetite, and maintenance for life—you can go to many different sources. The nutrition clinic of your local hospital or public health department can offer advice. So, too, can your family doctor. You could also consult a responsible weight-control organization like Weight Watchers, being sure that its food program was developed under professional supervision. You do not have to be a nutrition expert to plan your own program, but in choosing the plan you should have the benefit of professional advice.

A Sample Menu for the Week

Medical authorities recommend that 35 percent of the calories in our daily diets should come from fat, 45 percent from carbohydrates, and 20 percent from protein.[6] Fats are our most concentrated source of energy. They also serve as carriers for certain vitamins and they contribute to the health of our blood, arteries, nerves, and skin.[7] We eat two kinds of fats. Saturated fatty acids are essential to our diets, but when we take in too many, we can suffer from the problem of unhealthy buildup of fats in our hearts and circulatory systems. Saturated fats are found in whole milk, butter, eggs, and the "hard" fat of red meats. Polyunsaturated fatty acids are also essential to our diets and they can be found in vegetable oils, nuts like almonds, pecans, and walnuts, and skim milk, among other sources. Our fat intake should be balanced between saturated and polyunsaturated fatty acids.

Carbohydrates are a source of energy and they help to regulate the metabolism of fats and protein. Carbohydrates come in three different forms. In one form they are simple sugars like those in honey and fruit, or so-called double or refined sugars. In another form they are starches found in grains. Their third form is cellulose, available in the skins of fruits and vegetables. Sugar is an energy source but when sugar is taken in, blood sugar levels rise. When the sugar intake has been utilized, the body feels a need for more sugar and so more and more sweet food is eaten. Starches are also an energy source but because they are chemically more complex than sugars, their digestion takes longer and they are therefore a slower acting energy supply. Cellulose is important because it provides bulk to our diets and bulk helps to regulate intestinal and bowel functions.

Some carbohydrates have been termed "empty calories." These include the refined sugars and starches that contain food energy but none of the vitamins, minerals, and trace elements that are essential to good

health. Other carbohydrates like fruits and vegetables
provide calories along with these health-sustaining
elements.

Protein is the building material of our muscles,
blood, skin, hair, nails, and organs. Aside from water,
it is the most plentiful material in our bodies. The
building blocks of protein are the twenty-two amino
acids. Few natural proteins like a single kind of meat,
fish, or poultry contain all of the amino acids that our
bodies need. Therefore we must build into our diet a
rich variety of proteins so that our amino acid needs are
met.

Unfortunately, foods that are high in protein are also
often high in saturated fat. Prime meat with marbleized
fat is a good example. Therefore, it is important to buy
the leanest meat possible and to trim the visible fat from
it. It is also important to include at least three to five
fish meals in your diet for the week; fish is a protein
source with a lesser amount of saturated fat. Poultry,
also high in protein, is low in saturated fat.

Figure 16.1 presents a *sample* seven-day menu plan
that might be reported by a member of a Weight
Watchers class. Notice that the basic allowances shown
are those for women, with additional allowances of certain foods for adolescents and men. The following
week, this member would be encouraged to follow set
guidelines learned in class for preparing a menu plan
with some different foods. This food plan:

- Does provide all of the essential nutrients;
- Does offer enough food to control hunger;
- Does provide sufficient variety so that food interest can
  be sustained; and
- Does offer a program that permits reeducation of
  lifelong eating habits.

This is the kind of plan that you must learn to develop
with professional assistance.

FIGURE 16.1

A Sample Seven-Day Menu Plan*

DAY 1

Morning Meal	Orange, 1 small *50*
	Cereal, ¾ ounce *100*
	Skim Milk, ½ cup *50*
	Coffee or tea *200*
	Men and Youth Add: 1 slice Bread

Midday Meal	Fish
	Women and Youth: 3–4 ounces *200*
	Men: 4–5 ounces *50*
	Salad Vegetables *140*
	Bread, 2 slices *30*
	Margarine, 1½ teaspoons
	Coffee or Tea
	Men and Youth Add: Pear, 1 small
	Youth Add: Skim Milk, 1 cup

Evening Meal	Meat
	Women and Youth: 3–4 ounces
	Men: 4–5 ounces
	Cooked Broccoli, ½ cup
	Salad Vegetables
	Vegetable Oil, 1½ teaspoons
	Cherries, 10 large
	Coffee or Tea
	Men and Youth Add: Bread, 1 slice
	Youth Add: Skim Milk, 1 cup

*Basic allowances are for women. Adjustments for Men and Youth are indicated. In addition to those shown, men and youth can add one or two fruit servings daily, and youth can add 8 fl. oz. of skim milk.

Sample 7-Day Menu Plan © Weight Watchers International, Inc., 1982

Snacks,	Banana, ½ medium; Plain Unflavored Yogurt,
at	¼ cup; Crisp Bread, ¾ ounce; Skim Milk, 1 cup
Planned	*Men and Youth Add: Banana, ½ medium*
Times	

DAY 2

Morning	Prunes, 3 medium
Meal	Egg, 1
	Bread, 1 slice
	Skim Milk, 1 cup
	Coffee or Tea

Midday	Poultry
Meal	*Women and Youth: 3–4 ounces*
	Men: 4–5 ounces
	Cooked Spinach, ½ cup
	Salad Vegetables
	Vegetable Oil, 1 teaspoon
	Skim Milk, 1 cup
	Coffee or Tea
	Men and Youth Add: Strawberries, 1 cup;
	Bread, 2 slices

Evening	Fish
Meal	*Women and Youth: 3–4 ounces*
	Men: 4–5 ounces
	Baked Potato, 4 ounces
	Margarine, 2 teaspoons
	Cooked Beets, ½ cup
	Salad Vegetables
	Apple, 1 small
	Coffee or Tea
	Men and Youth Add: Apple, 1 small
	Youth Add: Skim Milk, 1 cup

Snacks,	Cantaloupe, ½ small; Mixed Vegetable Juice, 1
at	cup
Planned	*Youth Add: Pear, 1 small; Skim Milk, 1 cup*
Times	

DAY 3

Morning Grapefruit, ½ medium
Meal   Cottage Cheese, ⅓ cup
         Bread, 1 slice
         Skim Milk, ½ cup
         Coffee or Tea
            Youth Add: Skim Milk, ½ cup

Midday   Fish
Meal   *Women and Youth: 3–4 ounces*
            Men: 4–5 ounces
         Salad Vegetables
         Vegetable Oil, 1½ teaspoons
         Bread, 1 slice
         Nectarine, 1 small
         Skim Milk, 1 cup
         Coffee or Tea
            Men and Youth Add: Bread, 1 slice

Evening Meat
Meal   *Women and Youth: 3–4 ounces*
            Men: 4–5 ounces
         Cooked Peas, ½ cup
         Cooked Carrots, ½ cup
         Salad Vegetables
         Bread, 1 slice
         Margarine, 1½ teaspoons
         Skim Milk, ½ cup
         Coffee or Tea
            Men and Youth Add: Peach, 1 medium;
            *   Bread, 1 slice*
            Youth Add: Skim Milk, ½ cup

Snacks, Tomato Juice, 1 cup; Plums, 2 medium
at   *Men and Youth Add: Pineapple, ¼ small*
Planned   *Youth Add: Skim Milk, 1 cup*
Times

DAY 4

Morning Meal	Honeydew Melon, 2-inch wedge
	Cereal, ¾ ounce
	Skim Milk, ½ cup
	Coffee or Tea
	   Youth Add: Honeydew Melon, 2-inch wedge;
	                   Skim Milk, ½ cup

Midday Meal	Liver
	   Women and Youth: 3–4 ounces
	   Men: 4–5 ounces
	Cooked Onion, ½ cup
	Salad Vegetables
	Vegetable Oil, 1½ teaspoons
	Graham Crackers, 2 (2½-inch squares)
	Skim Milk, 1 cup
	Coffee or Tea
	   Men and Youth Add: Banana, 1 medium;
	                   Bread, 1 slice

Evening Meal	Veal
	   Women and Youth: 3–4 ounces
	   Men: 4–5 ounces
	Cooked Whole-Kernel Corn, ½ cup
	Cooked Zucchini, ½ cup
	Salad Vegetables
	Mayonnaise, 1½ teaspoons
	Bread, 1 slice
	White Wine, 4 fluid ounces
	Blueberries, ½ cup
	Skim Milk, ½ cup
	Coffee or Tea
	   Youth Add: Skim Milk, ½ cup

Snacks, at Planned Times	Chicken Bouillon, ¾ cup; Apple, 1 small *Youth Add: Skim Milk, 1 cup*

DAY 5

Morning Meal	Strawberries, 1 cup Egg, 1 Bread, 1 slice Skim Milk, 1 cup Coffee or Tea

Midday Meal
Cottage Cheese, 2/3 cup
Salad Vegetables
Bread, 1 slice
Margarine, 1 teaspoon
Skim Milk, ½ cup
Coffee or Tea
  Men and Youth Add: Grapefruit, ½ medium;
                    Bread, 1 slice
  Youth Add: Skim Milk, ½ cup

Evening Meal
Fish
  Women and Youth: 3–4 ounces
  Men: 4–5 ounces
Cooked Butternut Squash, ½ cup
Cooked Broccoli, ½ cup
Salad Vegetables
Vegetable Oil, 2 teaspoons
Peach, 1 medium
Coffee or Tea
  Men and Youth Add: Bread, 1 slice
  Youth Add: Skim Milk, 1 cup

Snacks, at Planned Times
Mixed Vegetable Juice, 1 cup; Applesauce, ½ cup; Plain Unflavored Yogurt, ¼ cup

  Men and Youth Add: applesauce, ½ cup; Graham Crackers, 2 (2½-inch squares)
  Youth Add: Skim Milk, ½ cup

DAY 6

Morning
Meal
	Orange Juice, ½ cup
	Cereal, ¾ ounce
	Skim Milk, 1 cup
	Coffee or Tea
	    Men and Youth Add: Banana, 1 medium
	                      Bread, 1 slice

Midday
Meal
	Beef Bouillon, ¾ cup
	Eggs, 2
	Salad Vegetables
	Mayonnaise, 2 teaspoons
	Bread, 1 slice
	Flavored Low-Calorie Gelatin, ½ cup
	Coffee or Tea
	    Men and Youth Add: Graham Crackers,
	                    2 (2½-inch squares)
	    Youth Add: Skim Milk, 1 cup

Evening
Meal
	Meat
	    Women and Youth: 3–4 ounces
	    Men: 4–5 ounces
	Cooked Brussels Sprouts, ½ cup
	Cooked Carrots, ½ cup
	Bread, 1 slice
	Margarine, 1 teaspoon
	Rosé Wine, 4 fluid ounces
	Tangerine, 1 large
	Coffee or Tea
	    Youth Add: Skim Milk, 1 cup

Snacks, *at* *Planned* *Times*	Grapes, 20 small; Skim Milk, 1 cup; Graham Crackers, 2 (2½-inch squares) *Men and Youth Add: Grapes, 20 small*

DAY 7

Morning Meal	Tomato Juice, 1 cup
	Cheddar Cheese, 1 ounce
	Bread, 1 slice
	Coffee or Tea
	Men and Youth Add: Grapefruit, ½ medium
	Youth Add: Skim Milk, 1 cup

Morning Meal

Tomato Juice, 1 cup
Cheddar Cheese, 1 ounce
Bread, 1 slice
Coffee or Tea
   Men and Youth Add: Grapefruit, ½ medium
   Youth Add: Skim Milk, 1 cup

Midday Meal

Fish
   Women and Youth: 3–4 ounces
   Men: 4–5 ounces
Salad Vegetables
Vegetable Oil, 1½ teaspoons
Blueberries, ½ cup
Skim Milk, 1 cup
Coffee or Tea
   Men and Youth Add: Blueberries,
                    ½ cup; Bread, 1 slice

Evening Meal

Poultry
   Women and Youth: 3–4 ounces
   Men: 4–5 ounces
Cooked Cauliflower, ½ cup
Salad Vegetables
Vegetable Oil, 1½ teaspoons
Bread, 1 slice
Cantaloupe, ½ small
Coffee or Tea
   Youth Add: Skim Milk, 1 cup

Snacks, at Planned Times

Plain Popcorn, 2 cups, Skim Milk, 1 cup; Pear, 1 small
   Men and Youth Add: Apple, 1 small;
                     Saltines, 6

Monitoring What You Eat

Once you have decided on what you should eat, it is a good idea to monitor your success in following the program that you have selected. For some purposes, keeping a complete "diary" of your food intake is important. For example, many members of Weight Watchers classes record their eating during a complete week from time to time in order to receive feedback from their lecturer about the appropriateness of their food choices. In general, however, a simple "yes/no" record can give you a great deal of information, enough to plan successful changes in your efforts to manage what you eat.

Figure 16.2 provides a simple, useful record. Notice that it includes the same information about eating urges and behavior that you were asked to collect in Chapter 2 (Figure 2:1) but adds two additional columns.

In column 5 check:

"Yes" if you ate a food that is included in the food plan that you are following;
"No" if the food that you ate is *not* included in the food plan that you are following; and
"None" if you ate nothing at all.

In column 6 check:

"Yes" if you ate an allowable portion of the food that you selected;
"No" if you ate more than the allowable portion of the food that you selected; and
Leave blank if you did not eat during this hour.

If you eat nothing during any given hour, check the "None" box when the hour is over. If you eat something, check the "Yes" or "No" box for choice and for portion size *before* you eat the food that you have chosen. Research has shown that by doing your recording *before* you eat, you can provide yourself with one additional choice point and may give yourself a chance to stop your problem eating before it begins.[8] In this way, recording what you eat can help you to control your food intake and work toward improving your chances for success.

In evaluating information from the chart, it is important to make note of many different kinds of information, including the following:

1. How many hours on which days did you eat nothing at all?
2. How often did you manage to eat nothing even though your urge to eat was strong (e.g., "3" or "4")?
3. How many hours did you eat the correct portions of well-chosen foods?
4. How many hours did you choose the proper foods but choose portions that were a bit too generous?
5. How many hours did you choose the wrong foods and eat too much of these?

Data about your successes is *more* important than data about your mistakes. Use these data to build your confidence about your strengthening self-control. Data about your mistakes is information that you can use not as a cue for self-reproach but rather as a stimulus for creative action.

For example, if you learn that you make constructive food choices throughout the day, but have difficulty during the evenings, try to identify the daytime strengths that can help at night as well. If you find that you have difficulty in managing your eating with others but do very well alone, try to think of ways in which you change the social eating conditions so that you can make use of some of the strengths that you draw upon when you are alone.

Finally, it is very important to monitor portion size by weighing and/or measuring each serving. "Portion drift" poses a major threat to effective weight control. For example, adding 1 ounce of meat to the women's noon meal allowance of 3–4 ounces increases the calorie content of that serving by 25 to 33 percent, an addition of about 80 calories. A bit of further carelessness during the day can undermine the best of intentions, since as

FIGURE 16.2

Expanded Personal Self-Monitoring Chart

Circle Day	Sunday	Monday	Tuesday	Wednesday	Thursday	Friday	Saturday						
(1)		(2)		(3)			(4)		(5)			(6)	
Time		Level of Your Urge to Eat		Did You Eat?			Planned Action		Did You Choose an Allowable Food?			Did You Take The Proper Amount?	
				Yes	No				Yes	No		Yes	No
7:00–8:00													
8:00–9:00													
9:00–10:00													
10:00–11:00													
11:00–12:00													
12:00–1:00													
1:00–2:00													
2:00–3:00													
3:00–4:00													

Time											
4:00–5:00											
5:00–6:00											
6:00–7:00											
7:00–8:00											
8:00–9:00											
9:00–10:00											
10:00–11:00											
11:00–12:00											
12:00–1:00											
1:00–7:00											

many as 200 or more uncounted calories may slip into the day's menu.

Eating on the Run

These days, when working women and men hold down two or even more jobs, it is not surprising that most of us feel pressured to prepare meals quickly and to eat them just as fast. Time pressure is often used as an excuse to stray from adherence to a meal plan, but it is a lame excuse and sets the stage for problem eating. Whether at home or away, you can have reasonable meals if you are willing to make the extra small effort.

Few gourmet menus are adapted to the needs of the time-pressured homemaker—who can make a 20-ingredient, 33-step recipe in 30 minutes?—but virtually any cookbook can be a goldmine of "quick and easy" recipes. When you have a few minutes to spare, glance through the recipes and circle those that seem to require ten minutes of preparation time or less—not counting actual cooking time. With these at your fingertips, you can plan your meals in advance. This can be an enormous time saver, because it will eliminate hunting expeditions through your recipe files and enable you to buy the ingredients for an entire week's menus beforehand. Building convenience foods into your plan can provide further savings: For example, many frozen foods are quite acceptable meals in themselves, or can become delicious supplements to those parts of the meal that you cook yourself.

With a little extra planning, you can save additional time. First, if you organize your kitchen so that the utensils you need are within arm's reach, you can shave precious minutes off preparation time. For example, keep cooking utensils and spices within arm's reach of the stove, and storage containers stacked on a shelf a step away from the refrigerator. Knowing your week's menu in advance, you can also prepare things in bulk, saving portions for subsequent meals so that you do not have to dirty the same utensil twice: you can dice enough onions for the week, storing those not used immediately in an airtight jar in the refrigerator; you can make sufficient salad dressing for the entire week; even cut and washed salad greens remain fresh for at least two days. As a further measure, you can cook two or three times the amount of food that you need for certain meals, freezing the remainder in meal-sized portions for future use.

Wise use of appliances can also be a valuable timesaver. For example, it may be better to slice one onion with a knife than to use the food processor, which requires more time than it's worth to clean. On the other hand, when making vegetable soup or any dish requiring a lot of chopping, grinding, or pureeing, the processor is more effective. In the same way, blenders, convection heat ovens, and similar appliances can help you shift treasured minutes from preparing your meals to enjoying them.

Just as you can eat quickly and prudently at home, so too can you when you are out, but you will have to select from the menu with care. For example, did you know that a quick lunch of three pieces of fried chicken, mashed potatoes with gravy, a roll, and a 12-ounce soft drink rings up 1,100 calories? Or that a superburger with fries and a chocolate shake have 1,230 calories?

The lion's share of these calories comes in the form of fat, whether in the meat, through deep frying, or in the cheese and sauces that are added. Deep frying can triple the number of calories in a 3-ounce potato, boosting it from 60 calories if baked to 235 calories if french-fried; two pieces of fried chicken contain over 350 calories, compared with the 120 calories in skinless, broiled chicken. Therefore, if you do plan to eat in fast-food restaurants, try to find ones that will broil your hamburger on racks so that the fat can drip off, or broil instead of fry your chicken or fish. Many restaurants will do this for you, even though the service is not advertised. Even then, it is a good idea to remove the skin from the chicken and the breading from fish as a further calorie saver that has almost no impact upon the taste of the food.

Many fast-food restaurants are now adding salad bars. If you eat in one that does not have such a feature, you would do well to bring your own vegetables, such as carrots or celery, to eat with your entree to provide a healthful amount of fiber. You are also well advised to add no salt to your food and to avoid high-sodium condiments because many fast-food restaurants salt their food fairly heavily during its preparation. If you are hypertensive, sodium restriction is a life-saving must, but even if you are not, you will benefit from reduced consumption because of sodium's fluid-retention properties.

As you can see, with proper judgment and assertiveness you can even follow a healthful meal plan in a fast-food restaurant. For example, by ordering medium or small hamburgers, perhaps eating only half the roll, having a salad instead of french fries, and drinking juice, skim milk, coffee, or tea in place of a soft drink or a shake, you can go far toward your calorie-restriction goal.

IN A NUTSHELL

Many people look for magic in the pantry. They look for special foods that will "absorb the calories" from other foods that they eat. They look for one or two foods that meet all of their needs so that they do not have to make decisions about what to eat. They look for very light diets and depend upon pills to blunt their appetites, fool their bodies into believing that they got more food than they actually have, or disrupt the digestion and absorption of the foods that they eat. Or they look for the severest of diets to take pounds off fast. All of these are short-range solutions—if they are solutions at all.

If you do not satisfy your basic needs for food, you will have difficulty following a program and are not likely to lose much weight.

If you do not re-educate yourself to choose food wisely as you lose weight, you will have little hope of maintaining your weight loss.

Therefore you must look at your weight-loss program as a time of personal renewal. Eat enough to feel satisfied and teach yourself how to choose food wisely while you motivate yourself with weight loss. This is the only safe way for you to take pounds off and have a reasonably good chance to keep them off.

Once you have chosen the food plan that you will follow, keep a record of your efforts from time to time. Evaluate your successes so that you can learn how to build on your strengths, and learn what you can from your mistakes so that you can build plans for greater self-mastery as your skills develop.

CHAPTER 17

Setting Your Sights

MOST PEOPLE HAVE a goal weight in mind for themselves. Perhaps you remember how much you weighed when you last felt fit and looked trim. Or perhaps you have failed the mirror test (found those pounds you thought you'd lost), the belt test (gasped for breath when you closed the belt of your favorite pants or dress), or the pinch test (found too much meat when you took a pinch of your midriff), and then made a "guesstimate" of how much fat you saw or held. Believe it or not, there is a good chance that your guess is more right than wrong.

Despite decades of research on the subject, experts still seek a reliable and efficient means of evaluating weight.[1] Everyone who has ever stepped on a penny scale or been examined in a doctor's office is familiar with tables of weight by height and sex. Some of these tables show the average weight of people with different characteristics. Other tables show desirable weights— those measures of pounds per inch of person that insurance companies tell us correlate' with average or better life expectancy. The problem with both tables is that the average person is heavier than the insurance companies tell us he or she should be, and even many with desirable weights can actually be obese. For obesity is a condition that exists when people have more than a normal load of fat—about 20 percent of body weight for men, 30 percent for women. Unfortunately, weight and fat are not the same; for example, during World War II some navy recruiters were embarrassed to learn that they had rejected as too heavy some of the foremost football players of the day even though they had hardly an ounce of fat on their well-toned bodies.[2]

Tables 17.1 and 17.2 represent the best compromise that the Weight Watchers medical experts could find between average versus desirable weights, and between measures of bulk versus proportion of fat. Notice that for men and women, a range of weights is given for people of different ages and different heights. The charts are used at Weight Watchers classes in the following way:

1. Find the weight range for people of your sex, age, and height.
2. Plan to lose weight until you reach the upper limit of the range for people in the group to which you belong.
3. When you have reached this upper limit of your goal weight range, you can decide whether this weight is acceptable to you or whether you should go on losing some or all of the pounds that would bring you to the lower limit of your goal weight range.

It is not possible to pick an exact weight for yourself before you begin to lose weight. People differ in the proportions of their bodies that are made up of bone and muscle. If you have more of either, your most desirable weight may be a bit higher than would be true for others who have less bone and muscle but whose age and height are the same as yours.

If you have any doubt about how much you should weigh, it is a good idea for you to consult your family

Table 17.1

Weight Range for Men

Height Range Without Shoes	Age in Years				
	18	19–20	21–22	23–24	25 & Over
Feet Inches	Weight in Pounds				
5 0 (60)	109–122	110–133	112–135	114–137	115–138
5 1 (61)	112–126	113–136	115–138	117–140	118–141
5 2 (62)	115–130	116–139	118–140	120–142	121–144
5 3 (63)	118–135	119–143	121–145	123–147	124–148
5 4 (64)	120–145	122–147	124–149	126–151	127–152
5 5 (65)	124–149	125–151	127–153	129–155	130–156
5 6 (66)	128–154	129–156	131–158	133–160	134–161
5 7 (67)	132–159	133–161	134–163	136–165	138–166
5 8 (68)	135–163	136–165	138–167	140–169	142–170
5 9 (69)	140–165	141–169	142–171	144–173	146–174
5 10 (70)	143–170	144–173	146–175	148–178	150–179
5 11 (71)	147–177	148–179	150–181	152–183	154–184
6 0 (72)	151–180	152–184	154–186	156–188	158–189
6 1 (73)	155–187	156–189	158–190	160–193	162–194
6 2 (74)	160–192	161–194	163–196	165–198	167–199
6 3 (75)	165–198	166–199	168–201	170–203	172–204
6 4 (76)	170–202	171–204	173–206	175–208	177–209

© Weight Watchers International Inc., 1975

Table 17.2

Weight Range for Women

Height Range Without Shoes Feet Inches	Age in Years				
	18	19–20	21–22	23–24	25 & Over
	Weight in Pounds				
4 6 (54)	83–99	84–101	85–103	86–104	88–106
4 7 (55)	84–100	85–102	86–104	88–105	90–107
4 8 (56)	86–101	87–103	88–105	90–106	92–108
4 9 (57)	89–102	90–104	91–106	92–108	94–110
4 10 (58)	91–105	92–106	93–109	94–111	96–113
4 11 (59)	93–109	94–111	95–113	96–114	99–116
5 0 (60)	96–112	97–113	98–115	100–117	102–119
5 1 (61)	100–116	101–117	102–119	103–121	105–122
5 2 (62)	104–119	105–121	106–123	107–125	108–126
5 3 (63)	106–125	107–126	108–127	109–129	111–130
5 4 (64)	109–130	110–131	111–132	112–134	114–135
5 5 (65)	112–133	113–134	114–136	116–138	118–139
5 6 (66)	116–137	117–138	118–140	120–142	122–143
5 7 (67)	121–140	122–142	123–144	124–146	126–147
5 8 (68)	123–144	124–146	126–148	128–150	130–151
5 9 (69)	130–148	131–150	132–152	133–154	134–155
5 10 (70)	134–151	135–154	136–156	137–158	138–159
5 11 (71)	138–155	139–158	140–160	141–162	142–163
6 0 (72)	142–160	143–162	144–164	145–166	146–167
6 1 (73)	146–164	147–166	148–168	149–170	150–171
6 2 (74)	150–168	151–170	152–172	153–174	154–175

doctor. You can do this at the start of your efforts to lose weight, when you reach the upper limit of your goal weight range, or at any point before you reach the lower limit.

Putting Your Weight into Perspective

After you have established your starting weight, and know your goal weight, you should start a graph that you will use to keep your weight in a lifetime perspective. Figure 17.1 shows the graph that Mrs. Green had used. It will teach you some very important lessons about weight control.

Mrs. Green weighed 180 pounds on Day 1 of her weight-loss effort. She is thirty-eight years old and is five feet five inches tall, so her goal weight range is 118–139 pounds. Realizing that loss of one and one-half pounds per week would be optimal for her, she estimates that she should reach the upper limit of her goal weight in approximately twenty-eight weeks (180 − 138 = 42 ÷ 1.5 = 28). Therefore she counts twenty-eight weeks and makes a dot at 138 pounds. Now she draws a very light line from 180 to 138 to give her expected rate of loss.

On the same day during each of the next twenty-eight weeks, Mrs. Green weighs herself at the same time of day, wearing the same clothing, on the same scale. She then puts a dot opposite the number of pounds that is appropriate, in the column for the current week. Going to a class for her weekly weighing or sharing her chart with a relative or friend can help to build her motivation to persevere.

Notice that Mrs. Green's actual experience differs somewhat from the line of her expected rate of loss. *This is true for everyone: our bodies are not perfect machines and they respond with some irregularity.*

First, it is clear that she lost more than three and one-half pounds during each of the first three weeks. This is

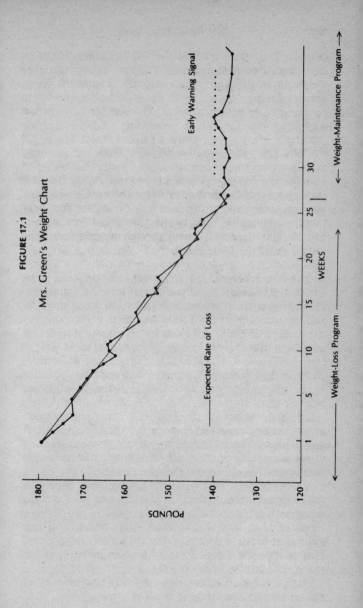

FIGURE 17.1

Mrs. Green's Weight Chart

Expected Rate of Loss

Early Warning Signal

POUNDS

WEEKS

←— Weight-Loss Program —→ ←— Weight-Maintenance Program —→

explained by the fact that she cut back her intake of carbohydrates (starches and sugars), eating some of these physically and psychologically important foods but consuming less than was her style before she began to change her eating patterns. Our bodies store excess carbohydrates for future processing and this storage takes place in a large amount of fluid. Water weighs 8.2 pounds per gallon and, when the extra starches and sugars are no longer consumed, the water that was used to store the old supply is voided by the body. It is this sudden loss of fluids that explains the initial rapid and very satisfying rate of loss that is not sustained for long.

After this initial fluid is lost, our bodies continue to lose weight irregularly even though we may eat food with almost the same number of calories one day after the next.[3]

There are several different explanations for these inevitable fluctuations in the rate of loss. All foods contain at least trace amounts of salt. On some days the sodium content of the foods we eat is higher than on other days. Because salt leads to the retention of fluids, more salt means more liquid, which means more weight. Another salt-fluid problem is experienced by women prior to their menstrual periods. Women begin to retain extra salt midway through their menstrual cycles, and the salt leads to the retention of extra water (which explains the "bloated" feelings that so many premenstrual women experience), with the fluids beginning to pass a day or two before the menstrual flow begins.[4]

Another cause of the predictable fluctuation in weight loss is any change in the reducer's level of physical activity. Remember that weight is gained when energy intake is greater than energy utilization, and weight is lost when we use more energy than we consume; any change in physical activity will have an effect when food consumption is fairly constant. Because many people tend to ignore physical activity as a factor in weight management, it would be wise to take a moment to consider what the scientists have taught us. A review of just two studies can set our thinking straight.

In the first study, a team of researchers at the University of Vermont made an attempt to have normal-weight young men gain weight by eating as much as three times their normal daily diet for periods of from three to five months. At the end of that time the men gained an average of only 10 percent of their body weight. But when the experiment was repeated in a prison setting, the inmate subjects gained as much as 25 percent of their body weight. The researchers concluded that restricted activity in the prison settings prevented the inmates from increasing their energy output to use up at least some of the extra calories, a feat that the lean subjects apparently accomplished as a means of keeping down their weight gain.[5]

The second study was the work of Dr. George Bray of the University of Southern California. He kept careful track of the food intake and energy output of patients participating in his weight-management program. As seen in Figure 17.2, his patients cut their energy utilization as soon as they reduced their caloric intake. In other words, when they started to take in fewer calories, they also began putting out fewer calories in the form of activity. The result was that *they undid much of the benefit they might have realized from their dietary efforts.*

Taken together, these studies show that many lean people gain weight slowly because they increase their activity in order to burn up the extra calories they consume. Heavy people, on the other hand, have a tendency to lose weight slowly because they cut down their activity in keeping with their reduced rate of energy consumption. In other words, when lean people consume more calories than their bodies need they seem spontaneously to increase the rate of their activity as a means of burning the extra calories rather than converting them to fat. Meanwhile, overweight people seem spontaneously to cut the rate of their activity when they eat less, making it more difficult for them to have a deficiency of the 3,500 calories which would allow them to lose each pound of fat. Knowing this can help weight-

FIGURE 17.2

Activity Rate and Caloric Intake

Among Weight-Losing Adult Women*

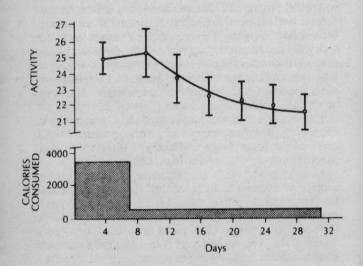

*Adapted from George A. Bray, Effect of caloric restriction on energy expenditure in obese patients, *Lancet*, 1968, *2*, 397–398.

conscious people to focus their attention on how much they do as well as on what they eat while trying to lose weight.

Any gains in weight which are occasioned by salt intake will be lost when the salt and resulting fluid retention are dissipated. This might take a matter of weeks. The scale might show no weight change whatever, despite the best possible eating discipline, because the scale cannot differentiate between fat and fluid. But eventually the fluids must be sloughed and a dramatic weight loss will vindicate the weeks of hard work. However, when the plateau in weight loss is due to inactivity, the body is left with a surfeit of calories that it can only handle by conversion into fat.

Weight losers are very sensitive to the numbers recorded on their scales. When a weight loss is expected and the scale shows a plateau or a small gain, the reducer can become discouraged and decide that the diet plan is not paying off. Discouragement such as this can lead to the abandonment of highly successful weight-loss programs. When the scale shows a weight gain in a week when the reducer knows that overeating *has* occurred, an effort should be made to analyze how to overcome the obstacle that produced the overeating. It is very important that the reducer avoid the trap of "catastrophizing," of deciding that all is lost because of overindulgence for a moment, a day, or even a week. Instead, it is important to apply the principles that have been learned to gain control of the troublesome situation.

It is also possible for a weight *loss* to occur during a week in which overeating has taken place. Many people take this as a sign that they can lose weight without paying strict attention to what they eat. Unfortunately, they are making a tremendous error, an error that often leads to dramatic and disappointing diet failures. Such weight loss following overeating should be considered a temporary and unearned parole, not a reprieve. Again, it is very important to analyze the circumstances that brought on problem eating and to take steps to develop a more effective self-control strategy for the future.

When weight has not been lost despite the fact that there has been no overeating during the week, this disappointing result must be understood as a common and by no means fatal occurrence. The weight loser should be comfortable with the knowledge that fat is being burned as long as food intake is reduced and activity levels are maintained. Therefore, a larger than normal weight loss can be anticipated a few weeks hence if the reducer merely continues to follow the weight-loss program. Look carefully at Figure 17.1 and you will see the peaks and valleys that brought joys and sorrows to

Mrs. Green as she worked on developing ever-higher levels of self-control.

Looking Ahead

Once Mrs. Green reached the upper level of her goal weight range, she felt that another ten-pound loss was needed. She persevered and lost those pounds, much as she expected. Then she entered a new phase of her weight-management program. She realized that her weight gains in the past always began one pound at a time. Even though she would have liked to think that she suddenly woke up one bleak morning twenty pounds heavier than when she had gone to bed, she had to reckon with the fact that this was never the case: she had had dozens of chances to reverse the process of weight gain before it got out of hand. Therefore, she decided to plan to keep her weight within a manageable range for the rest of her life.

Many people who succeed in maintaining the weight loss through monthly attendance at Weight Watchers classes do this very thing. A study of those who maintained and those who failed to maintain their losses led to the observation that *maintainers permitted themselves a very narrow channel of weight fluctuation while regainers waited longer to sound the warning bell.*

Those who maintained their losses felt that the time for action came when they strayed some two to five pounds above their goal. Regainers, on the other hand, did not believe that the time for action was upon them until their weights had risen twelve or more pounds. Unfortunately, the task of losing twelve pounds is far more formidable than that of losing five. Moreover, in the time that it took to gain back twelve pounds, many former bad habits could be strongly reestablished. For this reason, it is vitally important for you to add an *early warning system* to your weight chart. Then you will know it's time to act when taking action is still a

simple matter. On Mrs. Green's chart, the dotted line at
130 pounds is such a signal. Any time that her weight
moves above this warning line, she makes a special
effort to regain her self-control and in that way is never
far from her desired weight. Most people should work
within a range of from two to five pounds.

IN A NUTSHELL

It is important for you to have a goal weight, but to
realize that when you near your goal you may wish to
adjust your goal slightly down. It is also wise for you to
project the rate of your loss of weight, estimating your
losses at between one and two pounds per week. Be
prepared, however, to find greater losses at the beginning and plateaus or small gains once you are underway.
These are natural events that may be due to salt-fluid
retention or to changes in your rate of physical activity.
However, if you continue to follow your food plan as
you should, your fluid gains will eventually be lost. In
addition, if you regain your normal pattern of activity
after a brief rest brought on by illness, bad weather, or
the pressure of work, this plateau, too, can be overcome.

After you reach your goal weight, you will slowly be
able to add more food to your diet because you will no
longer need the caloric deficit that produced your
weight loss. These foods should be reintroduced slowly
and you should learn just how much you can add and
still maintain your weight.

Finally, when you do reach your goal weight, you
should establish for yourself an early warning system.
You should allow yourself a range of a few pounds
within which your weight will fluctuate, and you should
be ready to reestablish your weight-loss program whenever these limits are approached.

While you can add calories when you are at goal
weight, you must still be as careful in meal planning
during weight maintenance as you were during weight

loss. Whether you are striving to reach or to maintain
goal weight, you must be equally careful in managing
your eating behaviors. All of the techniques mentioned
in this book are useful in losing weight and in maintaining weight, and all should become your constant
companions throughout your weight-maintenance efforts.

CHAPTER 18

Is Weight Maintenance
Worth the Effort?

MANY PEOPLE CONCERN themselves with weight control only when they worry about how they will look in a bathing suit or when they struggle to shed enough pounds to fit into their party clothes. Once the summer sun has set or the party's over, they relax into their weight-gaining ways until the next cosmetic crisis. Unfortunately, this "yo-yo" pattern of weight gain and loss is as harmful to their health as to their egos.[1] The risks of carrying excess weight are so great as to make weight management anything but a matter to take lightly. If you are even just a little overweight, there is a good chance that you suffer in several different ways without your necessarily knowing what is happening.

Health Risks

The most obvious risks are the ways in which those extra pounds pose a burden for your health. Despite the fact that few of us believe that the worst could happen to us, the worst does, in fact, happen to an alarming number of men and women in the prime of their lives. For every 100 average-weight men who die in their twenties and thirties, only 72 underweight men will die young. On the other hand, as opposed to the 100 average-weight men, 141 moderately overweight and 212 severely overweight men will give up many of the best years of their lives.[2] Not very many of the seriously overweight escape life-shortening illnesses.[3] Men who are as little as 20 percent overweight have more than ten times the normal chance of becoming hypertensive. Hypertension, in turn, can lead to heart disease and death.[4] Diabetes is another life-shortening disease and one that can cause misery along the way. Overweight women have a 450 percent greater than normal chance of becoming diabetic, but their risk returns to normal when they lose their excess weight.[5]

Hypertension and diabetes are only two of the many illnesses associated with excess weight. The list also includes nephrosis or kidney disease, gout, premature ovarian failure, the shortness of breath which is known as the "Pickwickian syndrome" (named for the red-faced, bloated, gasping character from the Dickens novel), and crippling muscle and bone injuries brought on by saddling the hollow bones and thin muscle fibers with the need to support far more weight than they were designed to carry.[6]

Some very heavy people do manage to live out their lives without suffering from any of the common medical complications of obesity. But most overweight people suffer from at least some of these illnesses and they worry about falling victim to others. And for every overweight person who escapes physical ill effects, scores of others feel the effect of excess weight on their vigor and vitality.

Psychological Risks

If the health risks of obesity are pandemic, so, too, are the psychological risks. Because it is believed that fewer than one in twenty obesities involve identifiable physiological causes,[7] many researchers have tried to explain obesity as the result of psychological defects. For these researchers, some emotional problem is construed as the chicken, and those extra pounds are viewed as the egg.[8]

Early observations were dominated by the work of psychoanalytic writers who speculated that the obese have a personality defect arising from early life experiences.[9] However, hypotheses about rejecting mothers and children's turning to food for solace have not withstood the test of research. Moreover, it was learned that many events found in the families of the obese beset the lean as well.[10]

Later researchers tried to isolate some feature of the personalities of the obese that could account for their distress. Here again, any trait found among the obese was found in the lean as well, and the net result of decades of research has been the conclusion that the obese are *not more*—and may even *be less*—neurotic than the lean.[11]

There is, of course, the possibility that future research will show that the obese start life with a different emotional makeup from the lean. But the chances that any such difference will separate the tens of millions of the obese from the tens of millions of the lean is small indeed: psychology is just not that powerful and profound!

If there is no intrinsic psychological difference between the obese and the lean, how, then, can we explain the fact that the overweight are heavy without necessary physiological cause? The problem is *learning, not neurosis*. The overweight *learn* to eat more food than they need to keep themselves going and they *learn* to be less active than is desirable for their health and happiness. They learn other things as well: to surround themselves with the wrong kinds of food; to permit their eating to come under the control of many different kinds of environmental events that should have no relationship to food; to mismanage the timing and behavioral dynamics of their eating; to allow potential pleasures in their lives to remain untapped so that food plays too central a role; and to turn to food as a means of coping with troubling emotions.

The overweight are likely to have *less than normal stimulation* from social, vocational, and avocational activities, *more than normal self-consciousness* about food intake and body size, and *less than normal satisfaction* with what they achieve and how they manage their lives. Just as food is allowed to play too central a role in their active lives, so, too, do the overweight allow their management of eating to become *the* way that they evaluate their own performance as they go from day to day. This can lead to hypersensitivity, lessened self-satisfaction, and lowered productivity. Therefore, just as weight loss can help you to lead a longer and healthier life, it can also help you to lead a happier life as well.

Social Risks

The social risks of obesity are more subtle than the health and psychological risks. The social risks stem mainly from the stereotypes with which many people—fat and thin alike—regard the overweight.

Stereotypes are a convenience; they offer us prepackaged ideas about other individuals and groups without our having to expend the effort to form our own ideas. They are self-serving: they usually help us to feel good about ourselves, often at the expense of others. They are powerful because they guide our behavior toward others and thereby set up self-fulfilling prophesies. They are also pernicious because they often result in lost opportunities for our personal development and in cruelty toward others.

Most people have stereotyped ideas about themselves, their relatives, their friends and enemies, members of their church and of other churches, residents of their city, state, and country as opposed to those who live in other cities, states, and countries, people of their own race as opposed to those of other races, and people of their social class and occupation as opposed to those in other classes and occupations. Most people also have stereotyped beliefs about others who look different in some way. Some people tend to be suspicious, afraid, and at the same time condescending to those who have orthopedic handicaps, who are blind, or who show some outward sign of illness or injury. Unfortunately, even a little extra visible flab around the midsection can also trigger stereotyped reactions.

It has been found, for example, that overweight children are often rejected by their peers and do not receive equal treatment from their counselors at school: they are viewed as less capable than the lean. It has been found that college entrance officials tend to consider overweight applicants as less bright prospects than those whose weight is in the normal range. In the same vein, employers tend to expect light-weights to be better workers than heavyweights. Whether any of these expectations are true—and research does *not* bear them out—doors are often closed to the overweight, who only seek equal opportunity with the lean.[12]

Often without ever knowing the cause, the overweight experience prejudice at school, on the job, in the playground, and in every social situation. Their reaction can be disappointment and a turning against themselves; they feel that they have somehow brought about their own misfortune. To be painful, these experiences do not have to be gross: indeed, more subtle prejudice can cause the greatest level of self-questioning precisely because it is so difficult to pin down. Therefore the social risks of being overweight carry an importance equal to the risks of health and psychological weight-related stress.

IN A NUTSHELL

Even a few extra pounds can pose a more serious problem than you have realized. Extra weight may not be a direct cause of mortal illness. However, it has been shown to set the stage for some life-shortening illnesses and for other illnesses that can cause considerable discomfort. Overweight can also bring on psychological stress if you are confronted day in and day out with a tangible reminder that you failed to meet your own expectations. Finally, overweight can cause you to be closed out socially and it can prevent you from enjoying many of the opportunities that might otherwise be yours.

Weight control involves some work; it's not all play. But even the work brings with it the pleasure of achievement as you succeed in one objective after another. Moreover, the effort that you expend in learning how to manage your urge to eat can pay further dividends. You are learning ways to control your behavior in other areas of your life. When these dividends are added to the major benefit—reduction in the risks of being overweight—the reward for weight control is great indeed, and surely enough to justify a year-round effort.

CHAPTER 19

A Time to Meet the Challenge of Weight Maintenance

NOW THAT YOU have lost your excess weight and understand the health, psychological, and social reasons for keeping it off, it is time to gird yourself for the challenge of continuing to enjoy the new-found health and attractiveness of a slimmer you. Contrary to what many people believe, the maintenance of weight loss is not an easy matter; it requires realistic expectations, a set of new skills, and some contingency plans to use in the event that you begin to backslide despite your good intentions. As you do rise to meet this challenge, you can enjoy a renewed and realistic sense of self-confidence and know that you are capable of achieving any important goals that you set for the management of your own behavior.

What to Expect In The Months Ahead

Many people who suffer from the "yo-yo" syndrome have bought into the "dieter's delusion." This is a two-part self-deception. First, it is believed that the best route to weight loss is the fastest route, one that calls for eating so little of a narrow range of foods that hunger is constant and eating a bore. The goals of this diet are partly weight loss and partly self-punishment for having overeaten in the past. Next, it is believed that once weight is lost and the scales are balanced, it will be possible to return to former eating habits. Indeed, little else is possible when such a program is followed, because no new weight-control skills have been learned; and the likely outcome of reverting to old habits is of course the reexperiencing of old results—a loss followed by the insidious regain of weight that calls for moving into steadily larger sizes. Therefore, the first essential expectation for the period of weight maintenance is to

REALIZE THAT WHEN YOU REACH
YOUR DESIRED WEIGHT
YOU WILL FIND IT NECESSARY TO CONTINUE MANY
OF THE SKILLS THAT HELPED YOU LOSE WEIGHT,
AT THE SAME TIME ADDING NEW SKILLS
TO HELP MAINTAIN YOUR HARD-WON WEIGHT LOSS.

It is also important for you to realize that after weight loss you are essentially still the same person you were before, albeit lighter, healthier, and more attractive. This means you can expect to experience many of the same urges to overeat that you felt before; but if your weight-loss program has followed the principles out-lined in this book, those urges should be weaker and less frequent. On the positive side, you have a host of new coping skills. Unfortunately, however, many people panic when confronted by the first lust for chocolate chip cookies or freshly baked bread. Their panic springs from the fact that they associate this strong urge to eat large quantities of forbidden foods with their earlier failure to master the urge. The truth is, however, that while the urge may be the same, their ability to deal with the impulse is very different. While previously every wish may have become a reality, now each strong urge becomes an opportunity to reassert freshly learned self-management skills. Therefore, the second essential expectation for weight maintenance is the realization that

> YOU WILL UNDOUBTEDLY CONTINUE
> TO EXPERIENCE STRONG URGES
> TO EAT TOO MUCH OF THE WRONG FOODS
> ON OCCASION—EVERYONE DOES:
> BUT YOU HAVE A CHOICE
> AS TO WHETHER YOU YIELD TO THIS IMPULSE
> OR CONTROL IT.

Skills for Maintaining Weight Loss

With a new, more realistic set of expectations, you are ready to work on building the skills for maintaining your newly achieved shape.

Signal weight. Signal weight is the number of pounds that you feel you can safely gain above goal. As shown in Figure 17.1, it is extremely important that you draw a line on your weight chart to serve as an early warning signal for you to reinstitute your weight-loss program for a short time. Allowing your weight to drift above the signal level increases the challenge of reestablishing goal weight, because you will be required to restrict your eating for a longer period of time, and you will have allowed negative practices to strengthen poor eating habits.

Food planning. As you realize, you lose weight when your energy consumption falls below the level at which you use energy. The plan that you follow to lose weight drops your energy intake below the level at which you expend energy, so your body burns stored fat to keep itself going. (If you use fasting or another rapid-weight-loss method, your body may burn needed muscle and organ tissue as well as fat, so these programs should never be followed without the supervision of a physician.) Once you have reached the desired weight level, you will want to stabilize your weight by slowly increasing the amount of food you eat until you stop the weight-loss process. This means that week by week you should add from 50 to 75 calories to your daily meal plan until you find the level of food intake that allows you to maintain your weight *without weight gain*. For example, if you are a normally active woman of average height with some 50 pounds to lose, you probably followed a weight-loss diet that called for around 1,300 calories per day. This diet allowed you to lose about a pound each week overall. To maintain your current weight, you might try eating 1,350–1,375 calories each day for seven days. If your weight stabilizes at that level, then you have learned that you can maintain it on 1,350 calories. If you continue to lose, during the second week you might add another 50 to 75 calories, bringing your daily allowance to somewhere between 1,400 and 1,450 calories. You would then continue the process until you had experienced two weeks of weight gain. (Working with additions of only 50 to 75 calories per day, these gains should not exceed two pounds in total.) Then cut back to the calorie level you followed during the week before you had your first weight gain, and that becomes the level of your weight-maintenance food plan. As long as your activity level remains constant, you can safely stay at that level for the rest of your life.

If you followed a weight-loss food plan like the one illustrated in Chapter 16, you should have little difficulty in selecting foods for inclusion in your weight-maintenance program. In that plan you ate three meals plus one or two planned snacks daily. You chose an interesting variety of foods that were sufficient to keep your hunger under control and still meet your desire for a range of tastes and textures. You also chose foods that could become part of your normal weight-maintenance program. Having already developed skill in managing normal foods, all you need do to develop a weight-maintenance program is slowly to increase the size of the portions of the foods that you eat, or you may add one or more exchanges to the meal(s) of your choice. For example, if you decide to add 50 to 75 calories to your food plan for the first week, you might choose a second slice of toast for breakfast, or an extra vegetable serving at dinner. The second week, if you have the option of another 50-to-75 calorie addition, you might add an ounce of protein at your noon meal. As a general rule, if you wish to maintain nutritional balance, it is wise to add servings from different exchange lists—e.g., one fruit, one cereal, and one protein if you have the option of adding three servings.

As you prepare to add foods to your meal plan, there are two important things to bear in mind: First, many people who regain lost weight report that they never stray from eating the same foods consumed during weight reduction, and they wonder how they could possibly have suffered the return of lost weight. The answer can be found in a phenomenon called "portion-size drift." This occurs when weighing and measuring of portions ceases and standards become progressively more lax. Hamburger patties move from four to six ounces without notice, increasing their caloric value by half. Thin-sliced bread is exchanged for bread with thick slices, netting a 75-percent increase in calories. So too are the portions of butter, mayonnaise, pastas, beer or wine, and desserts gradually increased. Unfortunately, as portion sizes grow, so, inevitably will you. Therefore, it is essential to monitor carefully the quantity of each food you eat, not just for a little while but for the rest of your life. A second problem faced by many of those who struggle with weight maintenance is their desire to eat everything that they ever enjoyed consuming. You may have stopped eating certain foods that you found difficult to eat in small quantities (members of Weight Watchers classes learn to call these "red light" foods). Following weight loss, many successful maintainers find it useful to let sleeping dogs lie, and continue to omit these foods from their programs.

If you lost weight through a "quick weight-loss diet" in which you either ate very little, chose foods from a narrow list of selections, or even depended upon special prepackaged foods or food supplements, you will have a much more difficult time maintaining your weight loss. The main problem is that you lost weight without learning appropriate eating habits. It is unhealthy for you to continue your weight-loss program, and you must work to develop new habits without the reward of weight loss to spur you on. This is difficult, but by no means impossible. What you must do now is to start to follow a meal plan like the one illustrated in Chapter 16, and after two weeks of experience with it, gradually add food choices to the program until you reach a level of food intake that allows you to arrest the process of weight loss and achieve a comfortable level of weight maintenance.

Keeping your behavior in shape. Some important conclusions were reached about the behavior of maintainers versus regainers in the study of weight losers cited earlier. In addition to showing the effectiveness of a low signal weight, this research also demonstrated the fact that former members of Weight Watchers classes who continued to practice the self-management skills and physical activity program they learned in class were significantly less likely to regain weight. On the average, they were within five pounds of their goal weights 15 months after reaching goal, while their counterparts had regained over three times as much of their lost weight. Another key to successful weight maintenance certainly appears to be consistency in the eating and activity controls that were instrumental in promoting the initial loss of weight.

Here is a list of some of the techniques discussed in this book and also in Weight Watchers classes. Adherence to all of these steps can go far toward increasing the likelihood of successful weight maintenance.

1. Continue an optimistic, forward-looking approach to eating management.
2. Continue to think about yourself as a valuable person who has all of the needed assets for successful self-management.
3. Continue to make acceptable foods hard to find, while keeping problem foods out of the house.
4. Continue to eat at scheduled times and to extend the duration of mealtimes without increasing the quantity of food you eat.
5. Continue to manage your moods by changing situations that cause troubling feelings and by finding non-food-related ways of coping with problems that you cannot avoid.

Assuming that you will have to do more and not less to control your weight, and that you will continue to experience occasional strong urges to overeat, you should also

EXPECT TO HAVE STRONG DOUBTS ABOUT WHETHER WEIGHT CONTROL IS WORTH THE EFFORT.

In the last chapter you learned about the health, psychological, and social benefits of weight control. Awareness of these rewards is your ally in exercising self-control. Unfortunately, the benefits of good health, a sense of psychological well-being, and social acceptance are not always immediate, but rather are long-term outcomes. They are stacked up against the immediate appeal of some forbidden food, the feeling of being deprived and deserving a "pick-me-up," or perhaps the wish for prompt (albeit short-term) relief from feeling boredom, anger, loneliness, and worry. In this situation in which delayed benefits are matched against immediate rewards, choice of a positive alternative may require you to draw upon unusual resources—a challenge for which you can develop the necessary skills.

You should also

EXPECT TO EXPERIENCE SOME DISAPPOINTMENTS.

Many people who lose weight have unrealistic hopes and expectations, which are dashed after goal weight is reached. They may have looked to weight loss as a cure-all for various dissatisfactions in their personal lives—problems such as unhappy marriages or relationships, loneliness, or difficulties at work. With weight loss they expect to become a different person, figuratively and literally. They expect a new surge of satisfaction as those around them pay homage to all that they have achieved. There is a grain of truth in each of these expectations, insofar as they do open the door to new experiences. But none of these changes is automatic, and each requires some planned effort. To meet the challenge posed by all aspects of weight control as one element in successful living, it will be important for you to make a commitment to some new behavioral patterns that will serve you well:

6. Continue to ask for the constructive help of friends and family members.
7. Continue to build increased physical activity into your daily routine.
8. Continue to plan carefully what and how much you eat.

Why is it necessary to continue these practices? Because they are the keys to eating management, and without taking these actions that you know to be effective you allow yourself to fall prey to eating.

Continuing patterns of increased physical activity are as important as they were during initial weight loss. Activity helps to reduce appetite, to mellow troublesome moods, to condition your body, and to serve as a symbol for you and those around you that you are indeed in control of your own behavior. You may find it helpful to vary your activity routine; once you have lost weight you can select activities other than walking or stair-climbing. You might enjoy the occasional challenge of a competitive sport, a workout at a local health club, or a more vigorous solo activity, such as jumping rope. If you do try to perk up your interest in activity by choosing other options, please check with your doctor before you make any changes, just to be certain that you are making wise choices.

In addition to making continued use of the eating and activity management techniques that aided your loss of weight, you will also need some new skills for lasting weight control.

First, you will have to find a new important activity that can rival weight management as a focus of your attention. Successful weight loss requires careful planning and constant follow-through. People who work at weight reduction often weigh themselves daily, plan their days around their menus, read everything they can get their hands on about the latest "diet breakthrough," and discuss each diet triumph with friends who are ever willing to exchange similar tales. In other words, they have achieved the status of weight-control professionals, and weight change in either direction provides an opportunity to demonstrate their expertise. Whether gourmets or junk-food junkies, they know how to overeat, even if they do experience the pangs of guilt afterward. But they also know how to lose the weight once their largest clothes begin to feel too tight. Their weight-management efforts become the organizing principle of their lives, giving meaning to their days whether the number on the scale is heading up or down. For people with this affliction, nothing triggers interest or excitement as effectively as thoughts about what to eat or how to avoid eating a forbidden food.

If allowed to continue, this behavior paves the way for a lifetime of weight problems. The best way to overcome it is to find a new personal challenge that is powerful enough to replace weight control as a central concern. This new challenge should be something that

1. is very important to you;
2. can be shared or at least observed by others;
3. requires intelligence and thoughtfulness in planning, if not in execution;
4. requires some time for its achievement;

5. opens doors leading to new challenges; and
6. can be started immediately.

If it is unimportant, it will not offer sufficient motivation to sustain your interest. If it is an entirely private activity, you cannot receive the support of others. If it comes too easily, you will not have to think about it very much. If it is quickly achieved or is an end in itself, it will not outlast the appeal of the "yo-yo" game.

Listed below are several goals that various people have chosen as a means of ending their weight-control obsession and adding spice to their lives. In the blank next to each goal, write the numbers of the above-listed criteria that each goal fails to meet. If the goal passes the test, enter an asterisk in the blank.

___Carla's husband, Jim, would like her to learn to play bridge because it is a game that he enjoys very much. She thinks she'll give it a try because she knows Jim is not a good bridge player and she learns games quickly.

___Janie lives alone and has been concerned about the mess in her attic and basement for years. She thinks this is the time to tackle these chores.

___Jack has decided that he will finally devote time to building the stamp collection he has wanted to develop for years. He has been held back because he has not had time to study stamp values and learn about their history. Now that his youngest child has gone off to college, he feels that he has the time.

___Norm, Jack's son, lost weight with his father so he could go to school in slim, trim jeans. When school lets out in the spring and he is home for summer vacation, he plans to start to rebuild the antique car that his grandfather willed to him.

___Juliette has been a realtor for years. She has felt that some zoning ordinances are too strict, while others are too permissive. She would like to run for a seat on the county commission so that she can lend her knowledge to an effort to improve land use in her area.

Now that you have had your chance to evaluate these

goals, here's a chance for you to check your ratings in terms of the criteria listed earlier. Carla's goal falls short because it is not important to her (1), lacks intellectual challenge (3), and is too quickly achieved (4). It can be shared with others (2), would open the possibility of her making new friends (5), and could be started immediately (6). On balance, then, it is not a good choice. Janie's goal falls short because it is unlikely to attract the attention of others (2), can be achieved in a relatively short time (4), and creates no new opportunities (5). Even though it is important to her (1), may require careful planning (3), and can be started immediately (6), it is not a good choice.

Let's skip Jack for a moment and go on to Norm. His goal is important (1), can be shared with others (2), requires skill and intelligence (3) as well as considerable time (4), and could even be the foot in the door to a new career (5). Unfortunately, it fails the immediacy test (6), and Norm could regain the 60 pounds he lost before he loosened the first nut. Now we can look in on the last folks. Jack and Juliette are the bell-ringers in this exercise. Their goals meet all six criteria, and of the five people whose lives we have just shared, they are the two most likely to succeed in maintaining their weight losses.

Strange though it may seem, having a goal unrelated to weight may be the most important step that you can possibly take in maintaining your loss! Please take a few minutes now to start the process of choosing your goal. Begin by listing answers to the question, "What are some of the things you have wanted to do for some time that you can begin to work on now?" List six or more goals and then examine each one in light of the criteria that have been discussed. If none pass the test, list six more and keep at it until you reach the happy point at which you have chosen an objective appealing enough to command your attention and energy, and then begin working on your goal immediately; it's your first and best line of defense against undoing the good that you have done for yourself.

Another essential weight-management step calls for

learning how to act like a thin person. Once weight control is unseated as a major preoccupation and is replaced with a new source of excitement, it is necessary to take the next step into the world of the lean by developing action patterns similar to those chosen by thin people. This calls for some role playing in which you train yourself to think as if you were a comfortably thin person.[1] Making this shift will be easier for people who have lost a little versus a lot of weight, just as it is helpful if one has been overweight for a shorter rather than a longer time. It is also important for key people in one's social network to demonstrate some willingness to support rather than challenge newly emergent thin-action patterns.

To help clarify the difference between thought and action patterns of the obese and the lean, make your own decision about whether each of the ideas or behaviors in the list below is more likely to be observed in people who are overweight or lean.

More likely to be found in

	overweight	or	lean people
1. Thinking about oneself as lacking willpower.	____		____
2. Walking with a fairly distinct side-to-side movement.	____		____
3. Reading the dessert section of the menu before checking out the entrees.	____		____
4. Planning meals at the start of the day.	____		____
5. Looking for clothes first in the portly section of men's shops or in the size 24-or-over section of women's stores.	____		____

6. When looking in a mirror, concentrating on head and shoulders and avoiding looking at torso and legs.   ____   ____

7. At public gatherings, standing with back to the wall or placing pillow or purse on lap while sitting.   ____   ____

8. Skipping breakfast and following with a light lunch.   ____   ____

9. Double parking rather than finding a legal spot a block from one's destination.

10. Alternating between being very shy and retiring and being very pushy.   ____   ____

As you may have guessed, all but one of these actions are the benchmarks of the overweight. The sole exception is number 4: most weight-conscious lean people have a fairly accurate impression at the start of each day as to when, where, and how much they will eat during the day. In contrast, many overweight people do not plan their eating, but instead take things as they come. For example, they may "spontaneously" have a normal midafternoon snack, even though they might be going out for a celebration dinner that evening and expect to overeat a bit at the party.

Overweight people are more likely than the lean to give themselves negative behavioral promptings such as, "I'm the kind of person who always overeats," or "who never resists temptation." If they are fifty or more pounds overweight, they may have a tendency to walk with a swaying motion, to ignore their bodies while concentrating on their faces, or to try to hide body parts when in public. They often focus their attention on the very foods that pose the greatest eating-management challenge for them. They tend to reinforce a now outmoded "heavy" self-image by continuing to look at fashions for the overweight. They often omit planned meals when their self-control is strong, only to save their eating for the evening, when they have fewer supports for prudent eating. They often take energy-saving rather than energy-spending steps. Finally, they are frequently prone to rapid shifts in reaction patterns, because they often expect to suffer rejection on the basis of how they look rather than who they are.

You may experience some of these tendencies or none of them. You may do and think rather different things. Your thought and behavior patterns are as unique as your fingerprints. Therefore, you will have to write the script for your own thin role. Begin this process by making a list of all the thoughts and actions that you associate with being overweight. Check those that you think characterize your patterns. Opposite the items you have checked, write an alternative way of thinking or behaving. In a third column, list some thought and action patterns that you associate with being thin. Check those that you feel are presently lacking in your repertoire. The items written in column 2 (alternatives to overweight patterns) and the checked items in column 3 (thin patterns that are not normally yours) comprise the elements of your thin role.

Figure 19.1 offers an illustration of the lists prepared by one young woman. Please develop a chart like this for yourself and then spend at least 10 minutes studying it every morning until you have thoroughly learned your new role. While you are having your morning coffee, while you are sitting on the bus en route to work, or when you take your first rest break in the morning, read each item and visualize yourself acting in accordance with the role. After several weeks of practice, the elements in this thin role can become as natural to you as saying your own name, and you will have achieved another major advance toward mastering the skills you need to stay at your ideal weight for many years.

Planning for the worst. As a final plank in the platform of your development of new weight-maintenance techniques, it is time for you to learn how to deal with threats to your resolve before they occur.

Dr. Alan Marlatt[2] of the University of Washington has studied the tendency of people to suffer lapses in their self-control following their achievement of mastery over the urge to smoke, drink or gamble. His findings are also relevant to those pursuing long-term weight management. He found that most people feel comparatively confident about their ability to exercise willpower when they are flushed with the success of an initial hard-won victory. They then begin to experience a series of threats to their willpower. Among those whom he studied, Dr. Marlatt found that 35 percent of these threats took the form of negative emotional states, 20 percent took the form of social pressure, and 16 percent were experienced through interpersonal conflict. For the overeater, this would mean that moods such as boredom, depression, loneliness, or anxiety could lead to the urge to overeat, as could being pressured to eat too much of the wrong foods. Anger over minor conflicts in an important relationship can have the same result.

Research with different types of habit disorders has revealed three important truths about these challenges to self-mastery. It has been shown that the threat usually builds slowly in strength relative to the individual's sense of personal power. It has also been shown that the threats are more potent when the individual engages in an inner dialogue around the theme of personal weakness. Finally, vulnerability to such threats increases proportionately to the number of times in the past that temporary relief has been achieved through eating. These findings lead to three important rules:

1. MONITOR YOUR MOODS CAREFULLY. WHEN YOU REALIZE THAT A NEGATIVE FEELING IS BEGINNING TO BUILD UP, TAKE STEPS EITHER TO CHANGE THE SITUATION THAT IS ELICITING THAT FEELING, OR CHANGE THE WAY YOU LABEL THAT SITUATION.

FIGURE 19.1

Illustration of How to Formulate
a New "Thin Behavior" Role

Column 1 *Thoughts and Actions I Associate with Being Overweight*	Column 2 *Alternative to Column 1 Patterns That I Can Incorporate Into My New Thin Behavior Role*	Column 3 *Thoughts and Actions I Associate with Being Lean*	*Thin Patterns I Should Develop*
			—
Trying to joke and be funny all the time	Realize that there is more to me than my weight, and that I have worthwhile and interesting contributions to make	Not being self-conscious about weight or body size; concentrating more on others than on myself when I am with them	—
Not being selective about clothes; ignoring style and color and wearing drab, loose, tentlike clothes	Choose colors that look good on me and be aware of current fashions, choosing whatever I can that is new and fashionable but still appropriate for me.	Feeling in control of my body; engaging comfortably in many different physical activities	

Thinking that I look terrible anyway, so there's no point in experimenting with different hairstyles or making myself up more attractively	Get a more stylish haircut and "do"; experiment with different makeup to see what fits me best	Feeling secure within myself; not needing to please everyone else	___
Eating practically nothing all day, but grossly overeating at night	Have something interesting planned for every evening; find things to do that will take me out of the house	Wearing stylish clothes; being able to try all the latest fashions	___
Feeling so self-conscious about my size that I avoid activity for fear I might look ridiculous	Join an aerobic dance class and pay a month in advance so I will be forced to go; also, get in the habit of parking at least 2 blocks from work; use stairs instead of elevators	Being so engrossed in living that thoughts of food play a very minor part in my life	___
Hiding my body all the time behind plants, tables, other people, etc.	Be aware of my "hiding" patterns, and give myself messages that say: "Hey, that was the old you. Don't be afraid to show the world how you've changed—you look just fine!"	Good posture; moving in a proud way that tells the world I think I am okay.	___
		Being friendly and outgoing with others	___

2. WHENEVER YOU ARE AWARE THAT YOU HAVE BEEN TELLING YOURSELF THAT YOU PROBABLY HAVE LITTLE WILLPOWER, IMMEDIATELY CHANGE THE THOUGHT TO ONE THAT FOCUSES ON YOUR STRENGTH OR RESOLVE.

3. NEVER ALLOW YOURSELF TO HAVE A SNACK (OR A SMOKE OR A DRINK) WHEN YOU FEEL YOU MUST TO CONTROL A MOOD.

To comply with the first rule, you need only use a chart like that in Figure 2.1, replacing the "Urge to Eat" column with one reading "Strong Negative Emotion." Rate your moods on a five-point scale in which each number has the following meaning:

5 = feeling on top of the world
4 = feeling very good
3 = neutral feelings; not good, but not bad
2 = feeling pretty down, bored, worried, or angry
1 = feeling very down, bored, worried, or angry

As soon as you find yourself moving through 3 toward 2 or 1 on the scale, take some action to manage the troublesome situation *immediately,* using the techniques outlined in Chapter 11.

Meet the challenge of the second rule by reviewing the techniques and recommendations offered in Chapter 4. In this regard, it is important to remember that in large measure your behavior will conform to the expectations that you set for yourself. If you build a positive outlook toward your actions, you are likely to do things of which you will be proud. On the other hand, if you develop a negative attitude, you will be setting the stage for negative actions. Placing emphasis on your positive potential is essential.

You may have noticed that the third rule is stated negatively; it is the only "don't do" statement in this book. The negative statement is included for emphasis, because eating when your worries are high or your spirits are low may be the cardinal sin of weight control.

Once you reward yourself (yes, reward!) with food for having these troubling feelings, minor experiences of these emotions are likely to trigger a major urge to eat. You may even allow negative feelings to build in some measure in order to justify a snack or two. Therefore, it is important to assess your mood on the five-point scale offered earlier, and to confine all off-plan eating to those times when your mood rating is 3 or above.

These three rules will help bolster your willpower, but there will still be times when threats seem unmanageable. For example, when Mary overslept, spilled breakfast coffee on her dress, had a flat tire en route to work, and forgot her briefcase, she felt she deserved a treat at the office party, so she had quite a few—to her later regret. Harold had managed his weight quite well for weeks. When his twin sons came home for a college vacation, his wife made all of their favorite foods, which were of course also his favorites. Each time he entered the kitchen he was greeted by the aroma of freshly baked bread, or a dish of chocolate-chip cookies caught his eye. He managed to avoid these tender traps for the first week, but when he returned from a two-day business trip during which he had gotten very little sleep, his willpower seemed to be as fatigued as his body. He told himself that he was tired and therefore ought to have a snack. Both of these situations have something in common: both Mary and Harold fell into the trap of making what Dr. Lee Beach of the University of Washington[3] has called "Apparently Irrelevant Decisions" or "AIDs."

An AID is a bit of loose thinking that we use to make it easier for us to do things we know we should avoid, but would nevertheless like to do. Mary and Harold both wanted some snack food; Mary rationalized snacking because her day had begun badly, and Harold used his fatigue as an excuse. But flat tires and hectic business trips have no actual relationship to food; indeed, both are irrelevant to eating unless we invite them into our thinking to grease the skids leading to the pantry or the fridge. Mary's rough morning and Harold's hectic pace are therefore good examples of Apparently Irrelevant Decisions, just as are cleaning your plate to solve the hunger problems in China, stocking the pantry with sweets in case guests drop in, and deciding that you should binge because you have strong feelings or are bored.

To counteract your tendency toward loose thinking involving AIDs, make a list of the irrelevancies that you know you have used more than once in the past; then treat them in the same way that you respond to faulty advertising claims as discussed in Chapter 5: Label the ploy; identify the fly in the ointment; and then give yourself the correct message. For example, Mary might have labeled her ploy as a "poor me" maneuver; she might realize that she is grasping at straws in an attempt to justify overeating; and she could tell herself that her troubles en route to work have nothing to do with her body's need for food. Or Harold might label his maneuver as his "I work so hard that I deserve something extra" ploy. He could recognize that he tends to equate hard work with fatigue and to assume that fatigue warrants overeating. He could then set himself straight with a reminder that the best way to get recognition for his work performance is through his paycheck; and the best way for him to cope with fatigue is through moderate exercise or a five-minute nap.

Dr. Marlatt, whose work was mentioned earlier, has offered a suggestion for coping with situations that test your eating controls. Rather than avoiding thinking about these challenges, as many of us do, he recommends that we intentionally imagine ourselves in difficult situations, going on to visualize successful mastery of each of these challenges. As an example, a nightmare situation for Julia would be a delay at an airport for several hours, with nothing interesting to read and a snack bar a few steps from the waiting area. In the past she has eaten as many as six sweet rolls during a two-hour wait. A similar threat for Tom occurs regularly on visits to his mother-in-law. He has never especially liked her and feels he must eat the goodies that she serves because he doesn't want to offend her.

Following Dr. Marlatt's advice, Julia should imagine herself marooned in an airport waiting for a flight that has been delayed for five hours because of bad weather. She should add to her misery by imagining that she checked her briefcase, expecting to nap during her flight, which was to last a total of three hours. Irritation, boredom, and fatigue all overwhelm her as she watches others snap up what are advertised as "freshly baked" (but probably two-day-old) goodies. She should even imagine herself walking toward the counter. Then she should see herself make a hard right turn for the newstand instead, and imagine herself buying a paperback, finding a seat in the lounge where the snack bar is not in view, and quickly becoming engrossed in a tale of international mystery and intrigue. In the same vein, Tom should visualize himself as the victim of forbidden foods in the outstretched hands of his mother-in-law. He should imagine himself thanking her warmly for trying to prepare foods that she knows he likes, then asking her to help him achieve the weight-loss goals he would like to reach within the next few months. As a concluding scene, he should visualize a shift in focus from food to a discussion of his new business venture, where her accounting background could be a great help.

In work with families who are struggling to cope with delinquent children, a similar visualization process has been used quite successfully.[4] Parents and their children are asked to participate in a series of "What if . . . ?" exercises. For example, "What if the parents break a promise to lend their son the family car on prom night?" or "What if the son arrives home two hours later than expected?" By rehearsing responses to these and similar situations, parents and teenagers can develop a ready repertoire of responses to prevent difficult situations from becoming major crises. As a weight maintainer, you need a comparable set of "What if . . . ?" strategies. In the space below, please list the most challenging situations you can imagine, and opposite each item describe the way you would most like to respond. Reread the list from time to time and add any new threats that have come to your attention.

What If Terrible Eating-Management Challenges Arise? How Will You Respond?

Challenge	The Way I Would Like to Respond

IN A NUTSHELL

There is no magic in the maintenance of weight loss. Keeping pounds off is as much a matter of skill and determination as is losing weight in the first place. Many people who reach their goal weight feel they have earned a well-deserved rest from weight-management routines, only to find themselves tipping the scales a few months later at their former heavy weights. Therefore, you must be willing to make a firm commitment to change your thought and action patterns if you are to realize the promise of staying thin. This will require you to have realistic expectations for the weight-maintenance period. For example, you will have to continue to follow many of the principles that guided your loss of weight, while also adding some new weight-maintenance behaviors; and you will have to accept the fact that weight loss is not a cure-all for everything that troubles you, but rather a condition that enables you to make rapid strides in your own behalf. One of the most important of these strides is the need for you to find a new focus for your daily life, something as important and interesting as weight management, but without its resulting preoccupation with food. It is also important for you to develop skills for coping with the inevitable crises that will occur when you face previously irresistible treats at times of low resistance. Freedom from the weight-gain/ weight-loss treadmill means sustaining your newly learned self-management behavior while finding areas of commitment unrelated to weight. Fortunately, this goal is within the reach of everyone who is willing to make the effort!

CHAPTER 20

There Is an Answer

YOU KNOW THE risks of staying heavy and you have made a choice to work at being thin. Throughout this book you have been shown methods to improve many different aspects of your behavior. Behind these lessons has been a simple basic assumption:

PEOPLE ARE OVERWEIGHT
BECAUSE THEY DO NOT KNOW
HOW TO STAY AT THEIR DESIRABLE WEIGHT.

Obesity therefore equals misinformation and misguidance, not necessarily genetic bad luck or a weak character.

Many people rely upon diets to turn their weight around. But knowing what to eat is only part of the answer. Indeed, most weight-conscious people have a reasonably good idea of what goes into a healthful, weight-controlling diet. Therefore, it is as important to learn how to follow a food plan as to learn which plan to follow. Any effective weight-management system must train you to change your eating behavior, so that your food intake is what it ought to be. But the system must go further: it must also train you to minimize your urge to eat so that you are not bombarded by constant thoughts of food. This requires changes in far-reaching aspects of your lifestyle.

Because many programs focus only on food and not behavior, or because they focus on behavior in the narrowest sense and do not reprogram the urge to eat, many suffer from the so-called dieters' depression. This is a reaction to weight loss that includes feelings of disorganization, unhappiness, and tension. The people in whom these feelings are strongest are usually those who have been removed from their natural surroundings for weight loss, who were unusually depressed and anxious at the outset, and who follow crash programs that offer little behavioral retraining.[1] Under these conditions, adverse reactions are precisely what one would expect.

On the other hand, when fairly stable people attempt to lose weight in their natural environments, by following moderate dietary restrictions in a program that includes reeducation, they enjoy weight loss and positive mood change as well.[2] As an example, member attending a random sample of Weight Watchers classes across North America were less happy than their typical neighbors before they began their weight-loss efforts. Within five weeks of experiencing new levels of self-management success, however, their tested mood reactions were *better* than the norm.[3] So it is safe to assume that as you achieve control over your urge to eat, you will take new pleasure in many other aspects of your life as well.

Lest the wrong impression be given, weight loss is not without its stress. All changes create a certain amount of uncertainty and anxiety. We all take comfort in familiar aspects of our behavior and our life situations. Changes in our actions or in our environments almost always lead to a certain level of discomfort. For example, accepting a promotion with a higher level of pay and more interesting work can be a mixed blessing. With the greater rewards will come increased responsibilities: it is not uncommon for a person to wonder whether he or she will measure up. A party where there are many strangers is likewise a mixed blessing: it offers a chance to meet new people, but it also brings the risk of being rejected or ignored.

In the same way, developing new eating patterns means an important change. We are accustomed to the ways in which we use food, sometimes as a crutch and other times as a stimulus. When starting out on a new program, the weight loser has no assurance that the new patterns will be as satisfying as the old. We also develop patterns of social interaction that are influenced by our bodily dimensions. A very heavy person, for example, may be excluded from certain kinds of social interactions. Weight loss can open new doors but behind any of the doorways is the potential for failure. Therefore, shedding extra pounds can mean walking away from a convenient rationalization for inactivity—for some, a risky venture.[4]

You can expect to experience some tension: this is a natural consequence of your effort to learn new behaviors. And there may be times when you will be uncertain what to do as you seek new ways to handle old situations that triggered eating in the past. At times like these you will need imagination and support. Imagination will help you to see solutions to problems that appear to be irresolvable. Support will help you to take the actions that are necessary.

What is the best way for you to assure success in losing weight and maintaining weight? Some people are self-starters: they have the ability to stand aside from their normal routines and to find innovative solutions to their problems. They are able to risk change to reach an important goal. With the suggestions in this book, they can make a new beginning.

Other people work well with a partner. They can pair up with a relative or friend and share the mutual process of self-discovery and change. They can follow through on these suggestions and adapt them to their specific needs.

Most of us, however, are reluctant to reach out for new ways to meet old challenges. And most of us cannot sustain our motivation to change for more than a short time. We know that the development of new behaviors is a long and difficult process and our best bet may be to secure the support of more than one other person.

Those who have trouble going it alone, and who value group support rather than the support of a single individual, turn to groups for help in losing weight. However, all groups are not alike, and the differences significantly affect the quality of the services that they offer. In many respects, Weight Watchers is the standard-setter for weight-loss groups and you would do well to find a group that offers each of the following services, all of which are included in the Weight Watchers approach:

1. A food plan developed under professional supervision so that you can be certain that your basic nutritional requirements will be met while you lose weight and work to maintain your loss;

2. A food plan that can be adapted to the various stages of weight control—initial loss, any plateau experienced during weight loss, and the maintenance of your loss—so that you have guidance in food choice as your needs change through the progress that you make;

3. A socially constructive and positive interaction during meetings so that you receive the kinds of encouragement that you need in taking each successive step toward greater self-management;

4. Meetings that are clearly structured so that you know from week to week exactly what you are expected to do in an effort to build your self-control;

5. A behavior-change program that helps you to alter many aspects of your eating-related behavior including the change of those aspects of your environment that contribute to overeating;

6. A private weigh-in so that you get independent feedback each week about your progress; and

7. An approach that is taught to you in a manner that helps

to build your understanding of the reasons behind each recommendation so that you can, if you wish, build upon the recommendations and personalize the program to meet many of your own needs.

As a helpful reminder of many of the changes that have been recommended, please refer to the chart below from time to time. It lists all of the suggestions that have been offered in this book, and it can be used in two ways: When a challenge to your willpower arises, scan the list for a technique that you might have forgotten but that might very well turn the tide to your advantage; and periodically, even when things are going well, re-read the list to identify steps you might have been skipping or to find actions that you can take before the need arises. The list is yours to use; let it serve as your constant friendly reminder. The numbers in parentheses refer to the pages where the technique was introduced.

1. Chart your eating urges to find times and situations that test your willpower. Plan to change as many as you can to weaken your urge to eat (p. 10).

2. Correct errors in your thinking; for example:
   a. incorrect ideas, arbitrary inferences;
   b. dichotomous thinking;
   c. magnification of errors and disregarding of positives;
   d. terminal thinking;
   e. reversed thinking;
   f. fatalism (p. 22).

3. Improve your planning skills (p. 30).

4. Reevaluate your body image (p. 34).

5. Build a positive self-image (p. 45).

6. Psych out food commercials (p. 55) and build your resistance to their impact (p. 60).

7. Build a good offensive technique in the supermarket by:
   a shopping as seldom as possible;
   b. shopping from a list;

    c. shopping when you are *not* hungry;
    d. avoiding aisles in which you have no planned purchases;
    e. shopping with a friend (p. 62).

8. Reduce temptation at home by:
    a. not buying problem foods;
    b. keeping foods out of sight or out of reach;
    c. keeping pleasantly busy (p. 67).

9. Reduce temptation in restaurants by:
    a. choosing restaurants that serve foods you should eat;
    b. ordering what you want without reading the menu;
    c. ordering first so other people's orders don't tempt you;
    d. removing condiments and rolls or keeping them out of reach (p. 68).

10. Make eating a pure experience by:
    a. eating in only one setting; and
    b. engaging in no other activities while you eat (p. 78).

11. Slow your rate of eating by:
    a. waiting two minutes before starting to eat;
    b. cutting your food into bite-size pieces;
    c. putting your utensils down between bites;
    d. chewing food slowly;
    e. conversing between swallows;
    f. being the last person to start each course (p. 86).

12. Eat at predetermined times each day (p. 91).

13. Control your sense of satiety by:
    a. planning a range of foods with different tastes and textures;
    b. beginning meals with a generous salad;
    c. serving food on 7-inch plates;
    d. serving "hotel" rather than "boardinghouse" style (p. 96).

14. Manage nighttime eating by:
    a. preparing small snacks of acceptable foods;
    b. curbing fluid consumption in the late afternoon and evening;

    c. waiting ten minutes before eating;

    d. turning on the light and eating in your normal setting, if you must snack. (p. 97).

15. Control problem moods by:

    a. evaluating the way you label problem situations;

    b. using a structured way to make decisions;

    c. following a problem-solving plan;

    d. acting assertively to change problem-causing situations;

    e. planning rest and relaxation breaks;

    f. learning to meditate and to relax deeply (p. 117).

16. Control fatigue by developing better sleep patterns through:

    a. going to bed at the same time each night;

    b. waking up at the same time each morning;

    c. avoiding naps;

    d. controlling fluid and stimulant intake;

    e. making sleep a "pure" experience;

    f. relaxing to help yourself fall asleep (p. 131).

17. Get help from family members by:

    a. setting positive examples;

    b. providing gentle reminders;

    c. attending to positive achievements and ignoring lapses; and

    d. redirecting others who offer problem foods (p. 146).

18. Plan to follow a program of physical activity by:

    a. building activity into the normal fabric of your day;

    b. dedicating regular times to walking or a similar activity (p. 166).

19. Control binges by:

    a. eating normal meals each day;

    b. relying on distraction or thought stopping to deflect your attention away from food;

    c. waiting ten minutes before eating;

    d. choosing nonpreferred food;

    e. taking the smallest possible quantities of food, returning for second helpings only if absolutely necessary;

    f. turning the page and going on as if the binge had never taken place (p. 176).

20. Choose a food plan that:
    a. promotes gradual weight loss;
    b. provides all minimum daily food requirements;
    c. provides enough to eat so that hunger is avoided;
    d. provides variety of tastes and textures;
    e. allows you to learn new eating habits that you can maintain for life (p. 183).

21. Prepare a long-term graph of changes in your weight (p. 206).

22. Maintain your weight loss by:
    a. remaining optimistic about eating management;
    b. continuing to think of yourself as valuable and self-reliant;
    c. keeping problem foods out of the house, and non-problem foods hard to find;
    d. continuing to preplan and lengthen mealtimes, without increasing how much you eat;
    e. continuing to control your moods by changing your environment or by coping in non-food-related ways;
    f. asking for help;
    g. building and maintaining physical fitness;
    h. always planning your eating ahead of time (p. 223).

Whether you go it alone, choose a partner, or join a responsible group, you are starting out on a new road that leads to self-discovery and new ways to manage your behavior. Treat each challenge that you face as an opportunity for new learning. Meet each challenge through a series of small, well-chosen steps. Realize that for every challenge you face, you must choose one strategy that will help you break the behavior chain at a very early link, and a second strategy to call upon if the first fails to meet the test. Finally, be willing to hold nothing above the realm of change—be ready to change wherever change is needed. Do these things, and the joy of self-control awaits you!

Notes

Chapter 1

1. A. P. Burdon, Obesity: A review of the literature stressing the Psychosomatic approach, *Psychiatric Quarterly*, 1951, *25*, 568; R. I. F. Brown, The psychology of obesity, *Physiotherapy*, 1973, *59*, 216; A. J. Stunkard, Obesity and the denial of hunger, *Psychosomatic Medicine*, 1959, *21*, 282; A. J. Stunkard and S. Fox, The relationship of gastic motility and hunger: A summary of the evidence, *Psychosomatic Medicine*, 1971, *33*, 123; J. Hirsch, Discussion, *Advances in Psychosomatic Medicine* (Basel, Switzerland: Karger, 1972), *7*, 229; S. Lepkovsky, Fundamental problems of appetite control, in Nancy L. Wilson (ed.), *Obesity* (Philadelphia: F. A. Davis, 1969); D. J. McFarland, Recent developments in the study of feeding and drinking in animals, *Journal of Psychosomatic Research*, 1970, *14*, 229; N. E. Miller, C. J. Bailey, and J. A. F. Stevenson, Decreased 'hunger,' but increased food intake resulting from hypothamic lesions, *Science*, 1950, *112*, 256; O. W. Wooley, S. C. Wooley, and R. B. Dunham, Can calories be perceived and do they affect hunger in obese and nonobese humans? *Journal of Comparative and Physiological Psychology*, 1972, *80*, 250; P. T. Young, Physiologic factors regulating the feeding process, *American Journal of Clinical Nutrition*, 1957, *5*, 154.
2. See, too, G. R. Leon and K. Chamberlain, Emotional arousal, eating patterns, and body image as differential factors associated with varying success in maintaining weight loss, *Journal of Consulting and Clinical Psychology*, 1973, *40*, 474; and G. R. Leon and K. Chamberlain, Comparison of daily eating habits and emotional states of overweight persons successful or unsuccessful in maintaining a weight loss, *Journal of Consulting and Clinical Psychology*, 1973, *41*, 108.

Chapter 2

1. Daniel Cappon, Review article: Obesity. *Canadian Medical Journal*, 1958, *79*, 568.
2. J. E. Meyer and V. Pudel, Experimental studies on food intake, *Journal of Psychosomatic Research*, 1972, *16*, 305.
3. J. Rodin, Effects of distraction on performance of obese and normal subjects, *Journal of Comparative and Physiological Psychology*, 1973, *83*, 68.
4. O. W. Wooley and S. C. Wooley, Short term control of food intake, in G. Bray (ed.), *Obesity in perspective* (Washington, D.C.: U.S. Government Printing Office, 1975).
5. A. S. Bellack, R. Rozenský, and J. Schwartz, A comparison of two forms of self-monitoring in a behavioral weight reduction program, *Behavior Therapy*, 1974, *5*, 514; R. G. Romanczyk, Self-monitoring in the treatment of obesity: Parameters of reactivity, *Behavior Therapy*, 1974, *5,531;* R. B. Stuart, Behavioral control of overeating, *Behaviour Research and Therapy*, 1967, *5*, 357; R. B. Stuart, A three dimensional program of the control of overeating, *Behaviour Research and Therapy*, 1971, *9*, 177.

Chapter 3

1. W. H. Sebrell, Metabolic aspects of obesity: Facts, falacies and fables, *Metabolism*, 1957, *6*, 411.
2. Aaron T. Beck, *Cognitive Therapy and the Emotional Disorders* (New York: International Universities Press, 1962).
3. D. Meichenbaum, Toward a cognitive theory of self-control, in G. Schwartz and D. Shapiro (eds.), *Consciousness and self-Regulation: Advances in Research* (New York: Plenum Press, 1975).

Chapter 4

1. F. C. Shontz, Body image and its disorders, *International Journal of Psychiatry in Medicine*, 1974, *5*, 461.
2. John R. Buchanan, Five year psychoanalytic study of obesity, *American Journal of Psychoanalysis*, 1973, *33*, 30–35; A.

Stunkard and M. Mendelson, Disturbances of body image of some obese patients, *Journal of the American Dietetic Association*, 1961, *38*, 328; A. Stunkard and M. Mendelson, Obesity and the body image: I. Characteristics of disturbances in the body image of some obese persons, *American Journal of Psychiatry*, 1967, *123*, 364; A. Stunkard and V. Burt, Obesity and the body image: II. Age at onset of disturbances of body image, *American Journal of Psychiatry*, 1967, *123*, 1143.

3. P. F. Secord and S. M. Jourard, The appraisal of body cathexis: Body cathexis and self, *Journal of Consulting Psychology*, 1953, *17*, 343.

4. Myron L. Glucksman, Psychiatric observations on obesity, *Advances in Psychosomatic Medicine* (Basel, Switzerland: Karger, 1972), *7*, 194–216; M. L. Gluckman and J. Hirsch, The response of obese patients to weight reduction, *Psychosomatic Medicine*, 1969, *31*, 1–7.

5. P. Balch and A. W. Ross, Predicting success in weight reduction as a function of locus of control: A uni-dimensional and multi-dimensional approach, *Journal of Consulting and Clinical Psychology*, 1975, *43*, 119; D. W. Reid and E. E. Ware, Multi-dimensionality of internal versus external control: Addition of a third dimension and non-distinction of self versus others, *Canadian Journal of Behavioral Science*, 1974, *6*, 131; J. B. Rotter. Generalized expectancies for internal versus external control of reinforcement, *Psychological Monographs*, 1966, *80*, No. 1 (Whole No. 609).

6. V. Hays and K. J. Waddell, A self-reinforcing procedure for thought stopping, *Behavior Therapy*, 1976, *7*, 559.

Chapter 5

1. U.S. Bureau of the Census, *Statistical Abstract of the United States* (Washington, D.C.: U.S. Government Printing Office, 1975).

2. C. Lerza and M. Jacobson, *Food for People, Not for Profit* (New York: Ballantine, 1975), p. 165.

3. U.S. Bureau of the Census, *Statistical Abstract of the United States* (Washington, D.C.: U.S. Government Printing Office, 1975).

4. Ibid.

5. R. Choate, The sugar coated children's hour, in Lerza and Jacobson, *Food for People, Not for Profit*.

6. David M. Gardner, Deception in advertising: A conceptual approach, *Journal of Marketing*, *39*, 40–46.
7. U.S. Bureau of the Census, *Statistical Abstract of the United States* (Washington, D.C.: U.S. Government Printing Office, 1975).
8. G. Tom and M. Rucker, Fat, full and happy, *Journal of Personality and Social Psychology*, 1975, *32*, 76–766.
9. P. Taylor, Packaging: The costs add up, *Environmental Action*, August 10, 1974.

Chapter 6

1. R. E. Nisbett and S. Gurwitz, Weight, sex and the eating behavior of newborns, *Journ al of Comparative and Physiological Psychology*, 1970, *73*, 245.
2. S. Schachter and J. Rodin, *Obese Humans and Rats* (Washington, D.C.: Erlbaum/Halsted, 1974); D. Singh and S. Sikes, Role of past experience on food motivated behavior of obese humans, *Journal of Comparative and Physiological Psychology*, 1974, *86*, 503.
3. R. Goldman, M. Jaffa, and S. Schachter, Yom Kippur, Air France, dormitory food, and the eating behavior of obese and normal persons, *Journal of Personality and Social Psychology*, 1968, *10*, 117; L. S. Levitz, The susceptibility of human feeding behavior to external controls, in G. Bray (ed.), *Obesity in Perspective* (Washington, D.C.: U.S. Government Printing Office, 1975), p. 53; J. Mayer, L. Monello, and C. Seltzer, Hunger and satiety sensations in man, *Postgraduate Medicine*, 1965, *37*, 97; G. Tom and M. Rucker, Fat, full, and happy: Effects of food deprivation, external cues, and obesity on preference ratings, consumption, and buying intentions, *Journal of Personality and Social Psychology*, 1975, *32*, 761.
4. J. Rodin, Effects of distraction on performance of obese and normal subjects, *Journal of Comparative and Physiological Psychology*, 1973, *83*, 68; J. Rodin, The relationship between external responsiveness and the development and maintenance of obesity, in D. Novin, W. Wyrwicka, and G. Bray (eds.), *Hunger: Basic Mechanisms and Clinical Implications* (New York: Raven Press, 1976); P. Pliner, Effect of external cues on the thinking behavior of obese and normal subjects, *Journal of Abnormal Psychology*, 1973, *821*, 233.

Chapter 7

1. S. C. Wooley, Physiological versus cognitive factors in short term food regulation in obese and nonobese, *Psychosomatic Medicine*, 1972, *34*, 62.
2. A. M. Isen and P. F. Levin, Effect of feeling good on helping: Cookies and kindness, *Journal of Personality and Social Psychology*, 1972, *21*, 384; I. L. Janis, D. Kaye, and P. Kirschner, Facilitating effects of "eating-while-reading" on responsiveness to persuasive communications, *Journal of Personality and Social Psychology*, 1965, *1*, 181.

Chapter 8

1. S. W. Hill, Eating responses of humans during dinner meals, *Journal of Comparative and Physiological Psychology*, 1974, *86*, 652.
2. D. J. Gaul, W. E. Craighead, and M. J. Mahoney, Relationship between eating rates and obesity, *Journal of Consulting and Clinical Psychology*, 1975, *43*, 123; J. E. Meyer and V. Pudel, Experimental studies on food-intake in obese and normal weight subjects, *Journal of Psychosomatic Research*, 1972, *16*, 305; M. Wagner and M. I. Hewitt, Oral satiety in the obese and non-obese, *Journal of the American Dietetic Association*, 1975, *67*, 344.
3. A. R. Marston, P. London, L. Coiper, and N. Cohen, In vivo observation of the eating behaviour of obese and non-obese subjects, in A. Howard (ed.), *Recent Advances in Obesity Research*, vol. 1 (London: Newman Publishing Company, 1975).
4. O. W. Wooley, S. C. Wooley, and K. Turner, The effects of rate of consumption on appetite in the obese and non-obese, in A. Howard (ed.), *Recent Advances in Obesity Research*, vol. 1 (London: Newman Publishing Company, 1975), p. 212.
5. H. A. Jordon, Physiological control of food intake in man, in G. Bray (ed.), *Obesity in Perspective* (Washington, D.C.: U.S. Government Printing Office, 1975).

Chapter 9

1. G. G. Luce, *Biological Rhythms in Human and Animal Physiology* (New York: Dover Books, 1971).
2. H. Strughold, *Your Body Clock* (New York: Scribners, 1971).
3. S. Schachter and L. P. Gross, Manipulated time and eating behavior, *Journal of Personality and Social Psychology*, 1968, *10,* 98.
4. J. Rodin, Causes and consequences of time perception differences in overweight and normal people, *Journal of Personality and Social Psychology*, 1975, *31,* 898.
5. E. Wick, Overeating patterns found in overweight and obese patients, in M. E. Kline, L. L. Coleman, and E. K. Wick (eds.), *Obesity: Etiology, Treatment and Management* (Springfield, Ill.: Charles C. Thomas, 1974).
6. C. S. Chulouverakis, Facts and fancies in weight control: (1) Nibbling versus gorging, *Obesity and Bariatric Medicine*, 1975, *4,* 52.
7. G. A. Bray, Lipogenesis in human adipose tissue: some effects of nibbling and gorging, *Journal of Clinical Investigation*, 1972, *51,* 537; P. S. Wadhwa, E. A. Young, K. Schmidt, C. E. Elson, and D. Pringle, Metabolic consequences of feeding frequency in man, *American Journal of Clinical Nutrition*, 1973, *26,* 123; C. M. Young, D. L. Frankel, S. S. Scanlan, V. Simko, and L. Lutwak, Frequency of feeding, weight reduction, and nutrient utilization, *Journal of the American Dietetic Association*, 1971, *59,* 473.
8. P. Fabray, J. Fodor, Z. Hejl, and T. Braun, The frequency of meals: Its relationship to overweight, hypercholesterolemia and decreased glucose tolerance, *Lancet*, 1964, *2,* 614; F. Fabray, *Feeding Patterns and Nutritional Adaptations* (London: Butterworths, 1969); P. Fabray, J. Fodor, Z. Hejl, H. Geizerova, and O. Balcarova, Meal frequency and ischaemic heart-disease, *Lancet*, 1968, *2,* 190.
9. Editors, Feeding patterns in resistant obesity, *Food and Nutrition Notes and Reviews*, 1974, *31,* 34; J. F. Munro, D. A. Seaton, and L. J. P. Duncan, Treatment of 'refractory obesity' with a diet of five meals a day, *British Medical Journal*, 1966, *3,* 950; D. A. Seaton and L. J. P. Duncan, Treatment of 'refractory obesity' through a diet of two meals a day, *Lancet*, 1964, *2,* 612; C. M. Young, S. S. Scanlan, C. M. Topping, V. Simko, and L. Lutwak, Frequency of feeding, weight reduction, and body composition, *Journal of the American Dietetic Association*, 1971, *59,* 466.

Chapter 10

1. J. A. Brilat-Savarin, *The Physiology of Hunger* (New York: Dover, 1960).
2. S. Lepkovsky, Fundamental problems of appetite control, in N. L. Wilson (ed.), *Obesity* (Philadelphia: F. A. Davis, 1969).
3. P. H. Linton, M. Conley, C. Kuechenmeister, and H. McClusky, Satiety and obesity, *American Journal of Clinical Nutrition*, 1972, *25*, 386.
4. R. G. Campbell, S. A. Hashim, and T. V. Van Italie, Studies of food intake regulation in man, *New England Journal of Medicine*, 1972, *25*, 1402; J. M. Price and J. Grinker, Effects of degree of obesity, food deprivation, and palatability on eating behavior of humans, *Journal of Comparative and Physiological Psychology*, 1973, *85*, 265; H. A. Jordon, W. F. Wieland, S. P. Zebley, E. Stellar, and A. J. Stunkard, Direct measurement of food intake in man: A method of objective study of eating behavior, *Psychosomatic Medicine*, 1966, *28*, 836.
5. B. C. Walike, H. A. Jordon, and E. Stellar, Preloading and the regulation of food intake in man, *Journal of Comparative and Physiological Psychology*, 1969, *68*, 327; O. W. Wooley, S. C. Wooley, and R. B. Dunham, Can calories be perceived and do they affect hunger in obese and nonobese humans? *Journal of Comparative and Physiological Psychology*, 1972, *80*, 250; J. E. Meyer and V. Pudel, Experimental studies on food intake in obese and normal weight subjects, *Journal of Psychosomatic Research*, 1972, *16*, 305; O. W. Wooley and S. C. Wooley, The experimental psychology of obesity, in J. J. Silverstone (ed.), *Obesity: Pathogenesis and Management* (Acton, Mass.: Publishing Sciences Group, 1975); J. LeMagnen, Peripheral and systematic actions of food in the caloric regulation of intake, *Annals of the New York Academy of Science*, 1969, *157*, 1126; Henry A. Jordon, Physiological control of food intake in man, in G. Bray (ed.), *Obesity in Perspective* (Washington, D.C.: U.S. Government Printing Office, 1975).
6. A. J. Stunkard, Eating patterns and obesity, *Psychiatric Quarterly*, 1959, *33*, 284.
7. R. J. McKenna, Some effects of anxiety level and food cues on the eating behavior of obese and normal subjects: A comparison of the Schachterian and psychosomatic conceptions, *Journal of Personality and Social Psychology*, 1972, *22*, 311; S. Schachter and L. Gross, Eating and the manipulation of time, *Journal of Personality and Social Psychology*, 1968, *10*, 98.
8. G. G. Luce, *Biological Rhythms in Human and Animal*

Physiology (New York: Dover Books, 1971); J. M. Price and J. Grinker, Effects of degree of obesity, food deprivation and palatibility on eating behavior of humans, *Journal of Comparative and Physiological Psychology*, 1973, *85*, 265.

Chapter 11

1. G. A. Devos and A. E. Hippler, Cultural psychology: Comparative study of human behavior, in G. Lindzey and E. Aronson (eds.), *The Handbook of Social Psychology* (Reading, Mass.: Addison–Wesley 1969); S. Staurfer, A. Jundsain, R. Williams, M. Smith, I. Janis, S. Star, and L. Cottrell, Jr., *The American Soldier: Combat and Its Aftermath*, vol. 2 (Princeton, N.J.: Princeton University Press, 1949); E. J. Webb, R. Campbell, D. Schwartz, and L. Sechrest, *Unobtrusive Measures, Nonreactive Research in the Social Sciences* (Chicago: Rand McNally, 1966).

2. E. E. Abramson and R. A. Wunderlich, Anxiety, fear and eating: A test of the psychosomatic concept of obesity, *Journal of Abnormal Psychology*, 1972, *70*, 317; E. H. Conrad, Psychogenic Obesity: The Effects of Social Rejection Upon Hunger, Food Craving, Food Consumption, and the Drive-reduction Value of Eating for Obese vs. Normal Individuals (Ph.D. dissertation, New York University, 1969); C. P. Herman and J. Polivy, Anxiety, restraint and eating behavior, *Journal of Abnormal Psychology*, 1975, *84*, 666; J. McKenna, Some effects of anxiety level and food cues on the eating behavior of obese and normal subjects: A comparison of the Schachterian and psychosomatic conceptions, *Journal of Personality and Social Psychology*, 1972, *22*, 311; S. Schachter, R. Goldman, and A. Gordon, Effects of fear, food deprivation, and obesity on eating, *Journal of Personality and Social Psychology*, 1968, *10*, 91.

3. A. J. Lange and P. Jakubowski, *Responsible Assertive Behavior* (Champaign, Ill.: Research Press, 1976).

4. P. Jakubowski, A discrimination measure of assertion concepts (unpublished manuscript, University of Missouri, St. Louis, 1975; reproduced with the author's permission).

5. H. Benson, Your innate asset for combatting stress, *Harvard Business Review*, 1974, *52*, 49.

6. G. A. Marlatt and J. K. Marques, Meditation, self-control and alcohol use, in R. B. Stuart (ed.), *Behavioral Self-Management: Tactics and Outcomes* (New York: Brunner/Mazel, 1977).

7. D. J. Goleman and G. E. Schwartz, Meditation as an intervention in stress reactivity, *Journal of Consulting and Clinical Psychology*, 1976, *44*, 456; D. H. Shapiro and S. M. Zifferblatt, Zen meditation and behavioral self-control: Similarities, differences, and clinical applications, *American Psychologist*, 1976, *31*, 519; R. K. Walace and H. Benson, The physiology of meditation, *Scientific American*, 1972, *226*, 85.

8. J. Wolpe, *The Practice of Behavior Therapy*. (New York: Pergamon Press, 1969).

Chapter 12

1. I. Karacan, R. L. Williams, P. J. Salis, and C. J. Hursh, New approaches to the evaluation and treatment of insomnia, *Psychosomatics*, 1971, *12*, 81; A. McGie and S. M. Russel, The subjective assessment of normal sleep patterns, *Journal of Mental Science*, 1962, *108*, 642.

2. R. J. Berger, Bioenergetic functions of sleep and activity rhythms and their possible relevance to aging, *Federation Proceedings*, 1975, *34*, 97; W. B. Webb, Sleep as an adaptive response, *Perceptual and Motor Skills*, 1974, *38*, 1023.

3. L. C. Johnson, Are stages of sleep related to waking behavior? *American Scientist*, 1973, *61*, 326; M. A. Sackner, J. Landa, T. Forrest, and D. Greeneltch, Periodic sleep apnea, *Chest*, 1975, *67*, 164; J. M. Taub and R. J. Berger, Acute shifts in the sleep-wakefulness cycle: Effects of performance and mood, *Psychosomatic Medicine*, 1974, *36*, 164; W. B. Webb, Sleep behavior as a biorhythm, in W. P. Colquhoun (ed.), *Biological Rhythms and Human Performance* (New York: Academic Press, 1971); L. J. Monroe, Psychological and physiological differences between good and poor sleepers, *Journal of Abnormal Psychology*, 1967, *72*, 255.

4. J. M. Taub and R. J. Berger, Performance and mood following variations in the length of timing of sleep, *Psychophysiology*, 1973, *10*, 559; J. M. Taub and R. J. Berger, Acute shifts in the sleep-wakefulness cycle, loc. cit.; J. M. Taub and R. J. Berger, The effects of changing the phase and duration of sleep, *Journal of Experimental Psychology: Human Perception and Performance*, 1976, *2*, 30; J. M. Taub, P. E. Tangua, and D. Clarkson, Effects of daytime naps on performance and mood in a college student population, *Journal of Abnormal Psychology*, 1976, *85*, 210; R. T. Wilkinson, After effect of sleep deprivation, *Journal of Experimental Psychology*, 1973, *66*, 439.

5. M. W. Johns, T. J. A. Gay, J. P. Masterton, and D. W. Bruce,
   Relationship between sleep habits, adrenocortical activity and
   personality, *Psychosomatic Medicine*, 1971, *33*, 499; I.
   Karacan, R. L. Williams, R. C. Littell, and P. J. Salis, Insomniacs: Unpredictable and ideocyncratic sleepers, in *Sleep:*
   Physiology, Biochemistry, pharmacology, clinical implica-
   tions: First European Congress on Sleep research (Basel,
   Switzerland: Karger, 1973); I. Karacan, R. L. Williams, P. J.
   Salis, and C. J. Hursch, New approaches to the evaluation and
   treatment of insomnia, loc. cit.; L. J. Monroe, Psychological
   and physiological differences between good and poor sleepers,
   loc. cit.

6. R. D. Coursey, M. Buschbaum, and B. L. Frankel, Personality
   measures and evoked responses in chronic insomniacs, *Journal*
   of Abnormal Psychology, 1975, *84*, 239; W. C. Dement and C.
   Guilleminault, Sleep disorders: The state of the art, *Hospital*
   Practice, 1973, *8*, 57; S. N. Haynes, D. R. Follingstad, and W.
   T. McGowan, Insomnia: Sleep patterns and anxiety level,
   Journal of Psychosomatic Research, 1974, *18*, 69; A. McGhie,
   and S. M. Russell, The subjective assessment of normal sleep
   patterns, loc. cit.

7. A. H. Crisp and E. Stonehill, *Sleep, Nutrition and Mood* (New
   York: Wiley, 1976).

8. J. M. Taub, P. R. Tanguay, and D. Clarkson, Effects of
   daytime naps on performance and mood in a college student
   population, loc. cit.

9. A. H. Crisp and E. Stonehill, The relationship between weight
   change and sleep: A study of psychiatric outpatients, in *Sleep:*
   Physiology biochemistry, psychology, pharmacology, clinical
   implications: First European Congress on Sleep Research
   (Basel, Switzerland: Karger, 1973); A. H. Crisp and E. Stonehill, Sleep patterns, daytime activity, weight changes and psychiatric status: A study of three obese patients, *Journal of Psy-*
   chosomatic Research, 1970, *14*, 353; V. T. Karadzic,
   Physiological changes resulting from total sleep deprivation, in
   Sleep: Physiology, biochemistry, psychology, pharmacology,
   clinical implications: First European Congress on Sleep Re-
   search (Basel, Switzerland: Karger, 1973); P. Naitoh, R. O.
   Pasnau, and E. J. Kollar, Psychophysiological changes after
   prolonged deprivation of sleep, *Biological Psychiatry*, 1971, *3*,
   309; O. Petre-Quadens and J. D. Schlag, *Basic Sleep Mecha-*
   nisms (New York: Academic Press, 1971); M. A. Sackner, J.
   Landa, T. Forrest, and D. Greeneltch, Periodic sleep apnea,
   loc. cit.

10. G. S. Tune, Sleep and wakefulness in normal human adults,
    British Medical Journal, 1968, *2*, 269.

11. L. J. Monroe, Psychological and physiological differences between good and poor sleepers, loc. cit.

12. Ibid.

13. U. J. Javonovic, Suggestions for the treatment of sleep disturbances and conclusions, *Sleep: Physiology, biochemistry, psychology, pharmacology, clinical implications: First European Congress of Sleep Research* (Basel, Switzerland: Karger, 1973).

14. A. McGhie and S. M. Russel, The subjective assessment of normal sleep patterns, loc. cit.; R. Spiegel, A survey of insomnia in the San Francisco Bay area, cited in C. E. Thoresen, and T. J. Coates, Behavioral treatments for insomnia: A promise to be fulfilled, *Psychological Bulletin*, 1975, *83*, 340; I. Karacan, R. L. Williams, P. J. Salis, and C. J. Hursch, New approaches to the evaluation and treatment of insomnia, loc. cit.; I. Oswald, L. Adamson, and R. Norton, EEG, sleep and dependence studies of hypnotics, in *Sleep: Physiology, Biochemistry, Pharmacology, Clinical Implications: First European Congress on Sleep Research* (Basel, Switzerland: Karger, 1973).

15. F. Baekeland and R. Lansky, Exercise and sleep patterns in college athletes, *Perception and Motor Skills*, 1966, *23*, 1203; J. Hobson, Sleep after exercise, *Science*, 1968, *162*, 1503; J. Matsumoto, T. Hihisho, T. Suto, T. Sadahiro, and M. Miyoshi, Influence of fatigue on sleep, *Nature*, 1968, *218*, 177.

16. S. N. Haynes, D. R. Follingstad, and W. T. McGowan, Insomnia: Sleep patterns and anxiety level, loc. cit.; S. N. Haynes, M. G. Price, and J. B. Simons, Stimulus control treatment of insomnia, *Journal of Behavior Therapy and Experimental Psychiatry*, 1975, *6*, 279.

17. T. D. Borkovec and D. C. Fowles, Controlled investigation of effects of progressive and hypnotic relaxation on insomnia, *Journal of Abnormal Psychology*, 1973, *82*, 153; T. D. Borkovec and T. C. Weerts, Effects of progressive relaxation on sleep disturbance: An electroencephalographic evaluation, *Psychosomatic Medicine*, 1976, *33*, 173; J. H. Geer and E. S. Katkin, Treatment of insomnia using a variant of systematic desensitization, *Journal of Abnormal Psychology*, 1966, *71*, 161; E. Jacobson, *Progressive relaxation* (Chicago: University of Chicago Press, 1938).

18. R. D. Coursey, M. Buschbaum, and B. L. Frankel, Personality measures and evoked responses in chronic insomniacs, loc. cit.; D. Evans and I Bond, Reciprocal inhibition therapy and classical conditioning in the treatment of insomnia, *Behavior Research and Therapy*, 1969, *7*, 323; M. Kahn, B. Baker, and J. Weiss, Treatment of insomnia by relaxation training, *Journal of Abnormal Psychology*, 1968, *73*, 556.

Chapter 13

1. S. M. Garn, The origins of obesity, *Archives of American Journal of Diseases of Children*, 1976, *130*, 465; S. M. Garn and Dianne C. Clark, Trends in fatness and the origins of obesity, *Pediatrics*, 1976, *57*, 4431.

2. J. Bauer, *Institution and Disease* (New York: Gruen and Stratton, 1949); S. M. Garn and Dianne C. Clark, Trends in fatness and the origins of obesity, loc. cit.; Matsuki and Yoda, Familial occurrence of obesity: An observation about height and weight of college women and their parents, *Keio Journal of Medicine*, 1971, *20*, 135.

3. L. H. Newburgh, Obesity, *Archives of Internal Medicine*, 1942, *70*, 1033.

4. S. M. Garn, Personal Communication, June 24, 1976; Matsuki and Yoda, Familial occurrence of obesity, loc. cit.; R. H. Osborne and F. W. DeGeorge, *Genetic Basis of Morphological Variation* (Cambridge, Mass.: Harvard University Press, 1959); I. R. Shenker, V. Fisichelli, and J. Lang, Weight differences between foster infants of overweight and underweight foster mothers, *Journal of Pediatrics*, 1974, *84*, 715.

5. J. Hirsch, J. L. Knittle, and L. B. Salans, Cell lipid content and cell number in obese and nonobese human adipose tissue, *Journal of Clinical Investigation*, 1966, *45*, 1023; J. Hirsch, Adipose cellularity in relation to human obesity, *Advances in Internal Medicine*, 1971, *17*, 289; D. Brook, J. K. Lloyd, and O. H. Wolf, Relation between age of onset of obesity and size and number of adipose cells, *British Medical Journal*, 1972, *2*, 25; B. Salans, S. W. Cushman, and R. E. Weismann, Studies of human adipose tissue, *Journal of Clinical Investigation*, 1973, *52*, 929; P. Bjorntrop and L. Sjostrom, Number and size of adipose tissue fat cells in relation to metabolism in human obesity, *Metabolism*, 1971, *20*, 702.

6. R. D. G. Creery, Infantile overnutrition, *British Medical Journal*, 1972, *23*, 727; R. O. Fisch, M. K. Belek, and R. Ulstrom, Obesity and leanness at birth and their relationship to body habits in later childhood, *Pediatrics*, 1975, *56*, 521; A. G. L. Witelaw, The association of social class and sibling number with skinfold thickness in London schoolboys, *Human Biology*, 1971, *43*, 414.

7. T. R. Collins, Infantile obesity, *American Family Physician*, 1975, *11*, 162; L. S. Taitz, Overfeeding in infancy, *Proceedings of the Nutrition Society*, 1974, *33*, 113; Erica F. Wheeler, The problem of obesity in children, *Nursing Times*, 1972, *68*, 711.

8. R. L. Huenemann, Food habits of obese and nonobese adolescents, *Postgraduate Medicine*, 1972, *51*, 99.

9. S. L. Hammar, M. M. Campbell, V. A. Campbell, N. L. Moores, C. Sareen, F. J. Gareis, and B. Lucas, An interdisciplinary study of adolescent obesity, *Journal of Pediatrics*, 1972, *80*, 373; M. A. Hinton, E. S. Eppright, and H. Chadderdon, Eating behavior and dietary intake of girls 12 to 14 years old, *Journal of the American Dietetic Association*, 1963, *43*, 233; E. J. Kahn, Obesity in children: Identification of a group at risk in a New York ghetto, *Journal of Pediatrics*, 1970, *77*, 771; E. J. Stanley, H. H. Glaser, D. G. Levin, P. A. Adams, and I. L. Coley, Overcoming obesity in adolescents, *Clinical Pediatrics*, 1970, *9*, 29.

10. B. A. Bullen, R. B. Reed, and J. Mayer, Physical activity of obese and nonobese adolescent girls appraised by motion picture sampling, *American Journal of Clinical Nutrition*, 1964, *14*, 211; R. I. Huenemann, L. R. Shapiro, and M. C. Hampton, Teenagers' activities and attitudes toward activity, *Journal of the American Dietetic Association*, 1967, *51*, 433; M. L. Johnson, B. S. Burke, and J. Mayer, Relative importance of inactivity and overeating in the energy balance of obese high school girls, *American Journal of Clinical Nutrition*, 1956, *4*, 37; P. A. Stefanik, F. P. Heald, and J. Mayer, Caloric intake in relation to energy output of obese and non-obese adolescent boys, *American Journal of Clinical Nutrition*, 1959, *7*, 55.

11. P. A. Stefanik, F. P. Heald, and J. Mayer, Caloric intake in relation to energy output of obese and non-obese adolescent boys, loc. cit.; R. L. Huenemann, Food habits of obese and non-obese adolescents, *Postgraduate Medicine*, 1972, *51*, 99; J. B. G. A. Durnin, M. E. Lonergan, J. Good, and E. Ewan, A cross-sectional nutritional and anthropometric study, with an interval of 7 years on 611 adolescent school children, *British Journal of Nutrition*, 1974, *32*, 169; E. M. Hutson, N. L. Cohen, N. D. Hunke, R. C. Steinkamp, M. H. Rourke, and H. E. Walsh, Measures of body fat and related factors in normal adults, *Journal of the American Dietetic Association*, 1965, *47*, 179; M. C. McCarthy, Dietary and activity patterns of obese women in Trinidad, *Journal of the American Dietetic Association*, 1966, *48*, 33; G. A. Rose and R. T. Williams, Metabolic studies on large and small eaters, *British Journal of Nutrition*, 1961, *15*, 1.

12. S. Abraham and M. Nordsieck, Relationship of excess weight in children and adults, *Public Health Reports*, 1960, *75*, 263; F. P. Heald and M. A. Khan, Teenage obesity, *Pediatric Clinics of North America*, 1973, *20*, 807; J. K. Lloyd, O. H. Wolff, and W. S. Sheland, Childhood obesity: Long term studies of height and weight, *British Medical Journal*, 1961, *2*, 45.

13. F. P. Heald, Treatment of obesity in adolescence, *Postgraduate Medicine*, 1972, *51*, 109.

14. Richard B. Stuart and William J. Lederer, *Caring Days: Techniques for Improving Marriages* (New York: W. W. Norton, in press).

15. D. H. Karpowitz and F. Zeis, Personality and behavior differences of obese and non-obese adolescents, *Journal of Consulting and Clinical Psychology*, 1975, *43*, 886.

16. Richard B. Stuart and William J. Lederer, *Caring Days*.

17. L. S. Levitz, The susceptibility of human feeding behavior to external controls, in G. Bray (ed.), *Obesity in Perspective* (Washington, D.C., U.S. Government Printing Office, 1975).

Chapter 14

1. Food and Nutrition Board, National Research Council, *Recommended Dietary Allowances* (Washington, D.C.: National Academy of Sciences, 1974).

2. F. Konishi, Food energy equivalents of various activities, *Journal of the American Dietetic Association*, 1965, *46*, 186.

3. D. L. Costill and E. L. Fox, Energetics of marathon running, *Medicine and Science in Sports*, 1969, *1*, 81.

4. H. A. deVries and D. Gray, After effects of exercise upon resting metabolic rate, *Research Quarterly*, 1963, *34*, 314.

5. J. N. Morris, J. A. Heady, P. A. B. Raffle, C. G. Roberts, and J. W. Parks, Coronary heart disease and physical activity of work, *Lancet*, 1953, *2*, 1053; H. L. Taylor, E. Lepetar, A. Keys, W. Parlin, H. Blackborn, and T. Puchner, Death rates among physically active and sedentary employees of the railway industry, *American Journal of Public Health*, 1962, *52*, 1967; W. B. Kannel, P. Sorlie, and P. McNamara, The relation of physical activity to risk of coronary heart disease: The Framingham study, in O. A. Larson and R. O. Malmborg (eds.), *Coronary Heart and Physical Fitness* (Baltimore: University Park Press, 1971); E. R. Buskirk, Cardiovascular adaptation to physical effort in healthy men, in J. R. Naughton and H. R. Hellerstein (eds.), *Exercise Testing and Training in Coronary Heart Disease* (New York: Academic Press, 1973); S. M. Fox and J. L. Boyer, Physical activity and coronary heart disease, in H. H. Clarke (ed.), *Physical Fitness Research Digest* (Washington, D.C.: The President's Council on Physical Fitness and Sports, 1972); R. H. Rochelle, Blood plasma cholesterol changes during a physical training program, *Journal of Sports Medicine and Physical Fitness*, 1961, *1*, 63; H. L. Taylor, Relationship of physical activity to serum cholesterol

concentration, in F. F. Rosenbaum and E. L. Belknap (eds.), *Work and the Heart* (New York: Paul B. Hoeber, 1959); H. J. Montoye, Summary of research on the relationship of exercise to heart disease, *Journal of Sports Medicine and Physical Fitness*, 1962, *2*, 35.

6. S. Askanas et al., *Investigation into the effect of Medical Rehabilitation and of Therapeutic Procedure on Vocational Rehabilitation of Patients with Recent Myocardial Infarction* (Washington, D.C.: U.S. Department of Health, Education and Welfare, 1969); M. Cooper and K. H. Cooper, *Aerobics for Women* (New York: Bantam Books, 1972); D. C. Durbeck et al., The National Aeronautics and Space Administration–U.S. Public Health Service Evaluation and Enhancement Program, *American Journal of Cardiology*, 1972, *30*, 785; F. Heinzelmann, Social and psychological factors that influence the effectiveness of exercise programs, in J. R. Naughton and H. K. Hellerstein (eds.), *Exercise Testing and Exercise Training in Coronary Heart Disease* (New York: Academic Press, 1973); F. Heinzelmann and R. W. Bagley, Response to physical activity programs and the effects of health programs, *Public Health Reports*, 1970, *85*, 905; J. J. Kellerman et al., *Rehabilitation of Coronary Patients* (Washington, D.C.: U.S. Department of Health, Education and Welfare, 1969); R. B. Stuart, Exercise prescription in weight management: Advantages, techniques and obstacles, *Obesity and Bariatric Medicine*, 1975, *4*, 16.

7. Jean Mayer, *Overweight* (Englewood Cliffs, N.J.: Prentice-Hall, 1968).

8. H. K. Hellerstein et al., Principles of exercise prescription, in J. Naughton and H. K. Hellerstein (eds.), *Exercise Testing;* J. Naughton and R. Haider, Methods of exercise testing, in J. Naughton and H. K. Hellerstein (eds.), *Exercise Testing;* S. M. Fox, J. P. Naughton, and W. L. Haskell, Physical activity and the prevention of coronary heart disease, *Annals of Clinical Research*, 1971, *3*, 404; S. M. Fox, J. P. Naughton, and P. A. Gorman, Physical activity and cardiovascular health: III. The exercise prescription: Frequencies and type of activity, *Modern Concepts of Cardiovascular Disease*, 1972, *41*, 25.

9. B. J. Sharkey, *Physiology and Physical Activity* (New York: Harper & Row, 1975).

10. R. Passmore and J. V. G. A. Durnin, Human energy expenditure, *Physiology Review,* 1955, *35*, 801.

Chapter 15

1. J. Cautela, Behavioral therapy and self-control, in C. M. Franks (ed.), *Behavioral Therapy: Appraisal and Status* (New York: McGraw Hill, 1969).
2. K. Grinker, J. Hirsch, and D. V. Smith, Taste sensitivity and susceptibility to external influence in obese and normal weight subjects, *Journal of Personality and Social Psychology*, 1972, *22*, 320; J. A. Grinker, Obesity and taste: Sensory and cognitive factors in food intake, in G. Bray (ed.), *Obesity in Perspective* (Washington, D.C.: U.S. Government Printing Office, 1975), p. 73.
3. R. E. Nisbett, Taste, deprivation and weight determinants of eating behavior, *Journal of Personality and Social Psychology*, 1968, *10*, 107; J. M. Price and M. Grinker, The effects of degrees of obesity, food deprivation, and palatability on eating behavior of humans, *Journal of Comparative and Physiological Psychology*, 1973, *85*, 265; J. Rodin, Effects of obesity and set point on taste responsiveness and ingestion in humans, *Journal of Comparative and Physiological Psychology*, 1975, *89*, 1003.

Chapter 16

1. J. C. Gates, R. L. Hunenmann, and J. Brand, Food choices of obese and non-obese persons, *Journal of the American Dietetic Association*, 1975, *57*, 339.
2. B. A. Bullen, R. B. Reid, and J. Mayer, Physical activity of obese and nonobese adolescent girls appraised by motion picture sampling, *American Journal of Clinical Nutrition*, 1964, *14*, 211; R. B. Brandfield and J. Jordan, Energy expenditure of obese women during weight loss, *American Journal of Clinical Nutrition*, 1972, *25*, 971; R. J. Dorris and A. J. Stunkard Physical activity: Performance and attitudes of a group of obese women, *American Journal of Medical Science*, 1967, *233*, 622; A. M. Chirico and A. J. Stunkard, Physical activity and human obesity, *New England Journal of Medicine*, 1960, *263*, 935.
3. Walter M. Bortz, Predictability of weight loss, *Journal of the American Medical Association*, 1968, *204*, 99.
4. U.S. Public Health Service, *Obesity and Health* (Washington, D.C.: National Center for Chronic Disease Control, 1966).

5. J. F. Munro, Endocrine and metabolic disease: Obesity, *British Medical Journal*, 1976, *1*, 388.

6. W. H. Sebrell, *The Nutritional Adequacy of Reducing Diets* (New York: Weight Watchers International, 1977).

7. J. D. Kirschman, *Nutrition Alamanac* (Minneapolis: Nutrition Search, 1973).

8. A. S. Bellack, R. Rozencsky, and J. Schwartz, A comparison of two forms of self-monitoring in a behavioral weight reduction program, *Behavior Therapy*, 1974, *5*, 523.

Chapter 17

1. A. Keys, F. Fidanza, M. J. Jarvonen, N. Kimura, and H. L. Taylor, Indices of relative weight and obesity, *Journal of Chronic Disease*, 1972, *25*, 329; R. T. Benn, Some mathematical properties of weight-for-height indices used as measures of adiposity, *British Journal of Preventive Social Medicine*, 1971, *25*, 42; W. Z. Billewicz, W. F. F. Kensley, and A. M. Thomson, Indices of adiposity, *British Journal of Preventive Social Medicine*, 1967, *21*, 122; G. A. Bray, Types of human obesity, *Obesity and Bariatric Medicine*, 1973, *2*, 146; C. Seltzer and J. Mayer, A simple criterion of obesity, *Postgraduate Medicine*, 1965, A101; U.S. Department of Health, Education and Welfare, *Skinfolds body girths, biacromial diameter and selected anthropometric indices of adults* Washington, D.C.: U.S. Government Printing Office, 1970; S. M. Garn, The measurement of obesity, *Ecology of Food and Nutrition*, 1972, *1*, 333.

2. T. Gordon and Y. W. B. Kannel, The effects of overweight on cardiovascular diseases, *Geriatrics*, 1973, *28*, 80.

3. W. M. Bortz, A. Wroldson, P. Morris, and B. Issekutz, Fat, carbohydrate, salt, and weight loss, *American Journal of Clinical Nutrition*, 1967, *20*, 1104; T. R. E. H. Pilkington, V. M. Gainsborough, and M. Carey, Diet and weight reduction in the obese; *Lancet*, 1960, *1*, 856; T. Silverstone and T. Solomon, Long-term management of obesity in general practice, *British Journal of Clinical Practice*, 1965, *19*, 395; C. M. Young, N. S. Moore, K. Berresford, B. McK. Einset, and B. G. Waldner, The problem of the obese patient, *Journal of the American Dietetic Association*, 1966, *3*, 1111.

4. D. S. Janowsky, S. C. Berens, and J. M. Davis, Correlations between mood, weight, and electrolytes during the menstrual cycle: A reinantiotensin Aldosterone hypothesis of premenstrual tension, *Psychosomatic Medicine*, 1973, *35*, 143.

5. E. A. H. Sims, R. F. Goldman, C. M. Sluch, E. S. Horton, P. C. Kelleher, and D. W. Rowe, Experimental obesity in man, *Transactions of the Association of American Physicians*, 1968, *81*, 153.

Chapter 18

1. Surgeon General, *Obesity and Health* (Washington, D.C.: Department of Health, Education and Welfare, 1966).
2. D. Berkowitz, Obesity: Biological mechanisms, in L. Lasagna (ed.), *Obesity: Causes, Consequences and Treatment* (New York: Medcom Press, 1972).
3. G. V. Mann, The influence of obesity on health, Parts I and II, *New England Journal of Medicine*, 1974, *291*, 178, 226.
4. J. J. Alexander and K. L. Peterson, Cardiovascular effects of weight reduction, *Circulation*, 1972, *45*, 310; W. K. Kannel, N. Brand, and J. J. Skinner, Relation of adiposity to blood pressure and development of hypertension: Framingham study, *Annals of Internal Medicine*, 1967, *67*, 48.
5. J. H. Medalie, C. M. Papier, U. Goldbourt, and J. B. Herman, Major factors in the development of diabetes mellitus in 10,000 men, *Archives of Internal Medicine*, 1975, *135*, 811; T. D. R. Hockaday, Diabetes mellitus, *The Practitioner*, 1974, *213*, 535.
6. J. K. Alexander and K. L. Peterson, Cardiovascular effects of weight reduction, *Circulation*, 1972, *45*, 210; E. Fisher, R. Gregorio, T. Stephan, S. Nolan, and T. S. Danowski, Ovarian changes in women with morbid obesity, *Obstetrics and Gynecology*, 1974, *44*, 839; W. B. Kannel, N. Brand, and J. J. Skinner, Relation of adiposity to blood pressure and development of hypertension: Framingham study, *Annals of Internal Medicine*, 1967, *67*, 48; Massive obesity and nephrosis, *Nutrition Reviews*, 1975, *33*, 40; Respiratory complications of obesity, *British Medical Journal*, 1974, *2*, 519; A. Rimm, L. Werner, R. Bernstein, and B. Van Yserloo, Disease and obesity in 73,532 women, *Obesity and Bariatric Medicine*, 1972, *1*, 77; G. Tibblin, L. Wilhelmsen, and L. Werko, Risk factors in myocardial infarction and death due to ischemic heart disease and other causes, *American Journal of Cardiology*, 1973, *35*, 514.
7. H. I. Kaplan and H. S. Kaplan, The psychosomatic concept of obesity, *Journal of Nervous and Mental Disease*, 1957, *125*, 181.
8. L. Luborsky, J. P. Docherty, and S. Penick, Onset conditions

of psychosomatic symptoms: A comparative review of immediate observation with retrospective research, *Psychosomatic Medicine*, 1973, *35*, 187.

9. K. Abraham, The influence of oral erotism on character formation, in K. Abraham, *Selected Papers* (London: Hogarth Press, 1927); P. Burdon and L. Paul, Obesity: A review of the literature stressing the psychosomatic approach, *Psychiatric Quarterly*, 1951, *25*, 568; H. Bruch, *Eating Disorders: Obesity, Anorexia Nervosa and the Person Within* (New York: Basic Books, 1973); W. Hamburger, Emotional aspects of obesity, *Medical Clinics of North America*, March 1951, 483.

10. R. R. Keith and S. G. Vanderberg, Relation between orality and weight, *Psychological Reports*, 1974, *35*, 1205; R. A. Stewart, G. E. Powell, and S. J. Tutton, The oral character: Personality type stereotype, *Perceptual and Motor Skills*, 1973, *37*, 948.

11. L. P. Bronstein, S. Wexler, A. W. Brown, and L. J. Halpern, Obesity in childhood: Psychological studies *American Journal of Diseases of Children*, 1942, *63*, 238 (obese tended to be more intelligent); G. K. Gormanous and W. C. Lowe, Locus of control and obesity, *Psychological Reports*, 1975, *37*, 30 (I–E Scale did not differentiate); P. Balch and A. W. Ross, Predicting success in weight reduction as a function of locus of control: An unidimensional and ultidimensional approach, *Journal of Consulting and Clinical Psychology*, 1975, *43*, 119 (I–E Scale did differentiate); M. L. Held and D. L. Snow, MMPI, Internal-External Control, and problem check list scores of obese adolescent females, *Journal of Clinical Psychology*, 1973, *29*, 523 (MMPI did, but I–E did not differentiate); A. Kreze, M. Zelina, J. Juhas, and M. Garbara, Relationship between intelligence and relative prevalence of obesity, *Human Biology*, 1974, *46*, 109 (obese tended to have lower intelligence); R. Reivich, E. Ruiz, and R. Lapi, Extreme obesity, in N. Kiell (ed.), *The Psychology of Obesity* (Springfield, Ill.: Charles C. Thumas, 1975; no known MMPI profile for obesity); M. Rotmann and D. Becker, Traumatic situations in obesity, *Psychotherapy and Psychosomatics*, 1970, *18*, 372 (obese not more neurotic); J. Sallade, A comparison of the psychological adjustment of obese vs. non-obese children. *Journal of Psychosomatic Research*, 1973, *17*, 89 (obese children neither emotionally nor socially less well adjusted than nonobese); R. A. Wunderlich, Personality characteristics of super-obese persons as measured by the California Psychological Inventory, *Psychological Reports*, 1974, *35*, 1029 (C.P.I. did not differentiate); J. T. Silverstone, Psychosocial aspects of obesity, *Proceedings of the Royal Society of Medicine*, 1968, *61*, 371

(Cornell Medical Index showed obese not more neurotic than the lean).

12. N. Goodman, S. A. Richardson, S. M. Cornbusch, and A. H. Hastorf, Variant reactions to physical disabilities, *American Sociological Review*, 1963, *28*, 429; G. L. Maddox, K. Black, and V. Liederman, Overweight as social defiance and disability, *Journal of Health and Social Behavior*, 1968, *9*, 287; H. Canning and J. Mayer, Obesity: Its possible effect on college acceptance, *New England Journal of Medicine*, 1966, *275*, 1172; H. Canning and J. Mayer, Obesity: An influence of high school performance, *American Journal of Clinical Nutrition*, 1967, *40*, 352; D. Pargman, The incidence of obesity among college students, *Journal of School Health*, 1969, *29*, 621; K. T. Strongman and C. J. Hart, Stereotyped reactions to body build, *Psychological Reports*, 1968, *23*, 1175; G. H. Elder, Appearance and education in marriage mobility, *American Sociological Review*, 1969, *34*, 19; R. Straus, Public attitudes regarding problem drinking and problem eating, *Annals of the New York Academy of Science*, 1966, *133*, 792; G. L. Maddox and V. Liederman, Overweight as a social disability with medical implications, *Journal of Medical Education*, 1969, *44*, 214; J. Rodin and J. Slochower, Fat chance for a favor: Obese-normal differences in compliance and incidental learning, *Journal of Personality and Social Psychology*, 1974, *29*, 557; W. J. Cahnman, The stigma of obesity, *Sociological Quarterly*, 1968, *9*, 283; E. Goffman, *Stigma: Notes on the Management of Spoiled Identity* (Englewood Cliffs, N.J.: Prentice-Hall, 1963).

Chapter 19

1. R. B. Stuart, *Helping Couples Change* (New York: Guilford, 1980).
2. G. A. Marlatt, Relapse prevention: a self-control problem for the treatment of addictive behaviors, in R. B. Stuart (ed.), *Adherence, Generalization and Maintenance in Behavioral Medicine* (New York: Brunner/Mazel, 1982).
3. Dr. Lee Beach, University of Washington Department of Psychology; cited in G. A. Marlatt, above.
4. R. B. Stuart, T. Tripodi, S. Jayaratne, and D. Camburn, An experiment in social engineering in serving the families of delinquents, *Journal of Abnormal Child Psychology*, 1976, *4*, 243–261.

Chapter 20

1. H. Bruch, Psychological aspects of overeating and obesity, *Psychosomatics*, 1964, *5*, 269; C. V. Rowland, Psychotherapy of six hyperobese adults during total starvation, *Archives of General Psychiatry*, 1968, *18*, 541; A. J. Stunkard and J. Rush, Dieting and depression re-examined, *Annals of Internal Medicine*, 1974, *81*, 526; T. Robinson and H. Z. Winnik, Severe psychotic disturbances following crash diet weight loss, *Archives of General Psychiatry*, 1973, *29*, 559; A. J. Stunkard, The dieting depression, *American Journal of Medicine*, 1957, *23*, 77; D. W. Swanson and F. A. Dinello, Follow-up of patients treated for obesity, *Psychosomatic Medicine*, 1970, *32*, 209.

2. W. H. Biggers, Obesity, affective changes in the fasting patient, *Archives of General Psychiatry*, 1966, *14*, 218–221; E. Crumpton, D. B. Wine, and E. J. Drueick, Starvation: Stress or satisfaction? *Journal of the American Medical Association*, 1966, *196*, 394; W. G. Shipman and M. R. Plesset, Anxiety and depression in obese dieters, *Archives of General Psychiatry*, 1963, *8*, 26; R. I. F. Brown, The psychology of obesity, *Physiotherapy*, 1973, *59*, 216; G. G. Duncan, Correction and control of intractible obesity, *Journal of the American Medical Association*, 1962, *181, 309:* N. Fisher, Obesity, affect and therapeutic starvation, *Archives of General Psychiatry*, 1967, *17*, 227; J. T. Silverstone and B. D. Lascelles, Dieting and depression, *British Journal of Psychiatry*, 1966, *112*, 513; R. B. Stuart, The self-help approach to weight loss, in R. B. Stuart (ed.), *Behavioral Self-Management: Strategies and Outcomes* (New York: Brunner/Mazel, 1977); J. Grinker, J. Hirsch, and B. Levin, The affective responses of obese patients to weight reduction, *Psychosomatic Medicine*, 1973, *35*, 57.

3. R. B. Stuart, Sex differences in obesity, in E. Gomberg and V. Franks (eds.), *Gender & Psycho Pathology* (New York: Brunner/Mazel, in press).

4. E. V. Leckie and R. F. J. Withers, Obesity and depression, *Journal of Psychosomatic Research*, 1967, *11*, 107; W. G. Shipman and M. R. Plessett, Anxiety and depression in obese dieters, *Archives of General Psychiatry*, 1963, *8*, 530; J. T. Silverstone and T. Solomon, Psychiatric and somatic factors in the treatment of obesity, *Journal of Psychosomatic Research*, 1965, *9*, 249.

Index